Finally Finding My Voice

A true story from dying to thriving

Published in 2022 by Welford Publishing Copyright © Kate Fernandez 2022

ISBN: Paperback 978-1-7390970-8-0

Author photograph © Dearest Love 2022

Editor: Christine McPherson

Writing mentor: Cassandra Welford

A catalogue for this book is available from the British Library.

Finally Finding My Voice

A true story from dying to thriving

Kate Fernandez

For my girls
You fill my life with love and pride every single day

Contents

Introduction

My book has been written to share an insight into my healing journey – one which I have been on for most of my life.

There have been many occasions throughout my life when I could have given up completely, but I didn't. And I wholeheartedly believe that the main reason for this has been my family and friends who have supported me and challenged me at times.

I really hope that by reading my words, or listening to them, you will take away what you need to keep going on your own journey. You might find that some parts mean more to you than others, and that's fine.

Most of all, I want to pass on a positive, honest, and uplifting insight so that you can know that there is light at the end of what feels like a very, very dark tunnel at times.

It has taken me several years to get to this point of publication. At times, my head was fighting with my heart, but I was encouraged to write this mission statement by my writing mentor who told me it would help me to stay strong when the 'writing wobbles' kicked in. If you're reading these words in print then, along with my relentless determination, it worked!

Mission Statement

I am writing this book for myself to honour my life and my journey.

I am writing this book to help other people who may be on a cancer journey themselves or are supporting someone on their journey.

I am sharing my personal experiences, what I have learnt along the way about my body, and how to accept, love, and heal it.

I want to bring light into what can seem a very, very dark tunnel.

I am attracting readers who are open to hearing my story and who want to be inspired and uplifted with love.

This book is about the many chapters of my life. I will be sharing my truth from my heart in order to inspire others.

With love and gratitude,

Kate

Xxx

18th June, 2012

ENOUGH!!! I am in charge of what you do to me! I want to know what's happening!

I wanted to scream, but I couldn't make a sound.

My frustration reached boiling point as I ripped the feeding tube out of my nose. I couldn't take it anymore. I couldn't speak or swallow, let alone scream out loud. But I also couldn't stop the rage that had been building inside me for far too long.

I had endured 22 hours of surgery over two days, only to find out a few days later that I had a blockage in my neck which required yet another operation. That third visit to surgery was a turning point in my life! I felt with every bone in my body that I was incredibly lucky to have survived that trip to theatre, but made a conscious decision that when I did finally come around from the anaesthetic, enough was enough.

My entire life had consisted of me not speaking up, being scared of voicing my opinions, feeling like my voice didn't matter, or being very quickly silenced if what I was saying didn't want to be heard.

Now, here I was, literally, with no voice! It was in that very moment that I knew something had to change. I remember the look of horror on the nurses' faces as they tried to calm me down and reinsert the tube. They must have thought I had lost the plot. Despite being drugged up on copious amounts of pain relief and knowing that I had a long road of recovery, I also knew there were going to be big changes in my life. It was time for me to finally find my voice.

How had my life got to this point? And how did I break the relentless cycle of being seen and not heard?

Let's go back to the beginning…

Chapter: One

I was born at home in Crowle, which is a pretty little village on the outskirts of Worcester. I was my parents' first child, and I was much loved and cherished. My mum told me that she wouldn't put the vacuum round whilst I was sleeping, as she didn't want to disturb me.

I have happy memories of my early years, and I know from chatting with my mum that it was a time she remembered fondly. There were day trips out with her mother (my grandmother), with me in my pram (no car seats back then!) in the back of my mum's little red sports car.

Appearance meant a lot to my mum, and when I look back at old photographs of her, she was always dressed to impress. Her appearance mattered and was important throughout her life. The most stunning photograph I have of my mum was on her (first) wedding day in 1961. Mum looks almost regal and incredibly happy to be marrying her beloved John.

I will share more of my mum's story, I am sure, but she found it hard to go from living the high life in London and working with so many amazing people, to being simply 'Mum'. I think she felt trapped.

My parents worked in the licensed trade and kept various pubs and a restaurant during their married life. It was a way of life that I got used to as I grew up. There were many stories of big celebrations, staff disputes, and some memories that sounded more like scenes from *Fawlty Towers*! There were staff of all different nationalities, the majority being Italian and Spanish, and sometimes they just didn't get on!

The licensed trade is not a job; in my opinion, it's a way of life. And as my parents worked so hard, there were rare trips away and little time off.

Both my parents had worked in other industries. Dad had been in the Army, he trained as a metallurgist, concerned with the extraction and processing of various metals and alloys, investigating and examining their performance, and using them to produce a range of useful products and materials with certain properties. He also spent some time as an insurance salesman!

Mum had been a PA, secretary, children's nanny, had demonstrated cookers for Revo Electric (there is photographic evidence of this), and many other jobs besides. She could organise anything!

I don't think she had particularly enjoyed her school years, but both she and Dad were determined that they wanted to provide a good education for me and my little sister, so earning enough to provide a private education was high up on their list of priorities.

I have happy memories of attending a little prep school from the age of three, where I wore a beautiful blue uniform with a pleated skirt and blazer and boater hat. I liked school at that point, and my reports were simple and full of remarks like 'makes a good attempt' and 'tries hard and shows some improvement', but also 'I feel Kate could do a little better for her age'.

Then, when I was five, it was on to proper school – a private school in a beautiful old building, with amazing grounds, an outdoor swimming pool, netball courts, and a huge playing field. I can recall the beautiful curved, highly polished staircase, stunning tiled floors, huge classrooms, and long corridors. Sadly, though, this beautiful building has since been pulled down and replaced by houses.

From what I can remember, I worked hard but didn't feel very able or that learning came easy. I can remember learning Latin and never understanding why. All I can recall now is amo, amas, amat, amamus, amatis, amant, which I used to recite to myself. It translates as follows: *amo*: I love; *amas*: you love; *amat*: he, she, or it loves; amamus: we love; amatis: you (plural) love; amant: they love.

I particularly enjoyed drama at school, and remember taking part in a production of 'Joseph and the Amazing Technicolour Dreamcoat', and also 'Oliver'. To this day, music from both takes me right back to the stage at the end of the big hall.

There were several teachers who I can recall very clearly. Mrs Perks was a strong lady who taught all the PE. A hard taskmaster, she also coached the England netball team. Mrs Perks inspired my love of swimming, even though we learnt in a freezing cold outdoor pool. When you jumped in the water, it took your breath away, but somehow that was better than standing on the edge and very quickly turning blue after getting changed in the wooden huts at the end of the swimming pool.

When I was checking dates for this book, I saw a post about Mrs Perks, who sadly died last year. But I also found that she had been awarded an MBE, which didn't surprise me, as she inspired me and so many others.

There were a few high points at school, including the poetry competition when we were asked to recite our favourite poem. Mine at the time was by Pam Ayres, 'I Wish I'd Looked After My Teeth'. That choice of poem brings a smile to my face now, but you will find out why later in the book!

When I was five years old, my sister arrived. At that point, my parents were running an incredibly successful pub, and Mum gave birth and was back at work in the kitchen the next day! I have a vivid recollection from the summer of 1976, with trestle tables in the back garden of the pub, with barrels on and huge amounts of food. A balmy summer night, it was still light at 11pm, and there was an amazing atmosphere, which I think is why it sticks in my memory.

Life seemed to be good back then. There were such characters who came into the pub, including the jewellers from the Jewellery Quarter in Birmingham, and the car enthusiasts, and the darts teams; the list could go on and on! We lived above the pub, and I had to walk behind the main bar and top bar to head up the stairs to bed.

I can remember some of the regulars as if it were yesterday. I don't know if you remember 'The Muppets' TV show, which first aired in September 1976. One of the characters in the show would always sing 'Mahna, Mahna, Do Do Do', and as my sister and I passed through the bar, one of our regulars would sing it while some of the others would impersonate Kermit, Miss Piggy, and the other crazy characters. They provided such a sense of silliness and fun!

My parents worked incredibly hard and created a business they were proud of, but I remember one event that could have turned out very differently. A truck had parked on the hill opposite the pub. However, its brakes failed, and it came rushing down the hill towards the pub and the outside toilet block! Thankfully, it was moving fast enough that it took off and went over the top of the gents and landed in the back garden. Not much fun for the men in the gents, who saw a huge truck pass over their heads in broad daylight as they were standing there!

During our school summer holidays, we would spend time with my dad's parents. They had lived nearby but then retired to a tiny little hamlet near Worcester, buying a simple little bungalow with about an acre of land. I clearly remember spending many hours sitting at the kitchen table with my Nanna.

I remember my Grandad as being a very serious person who had worked hard for many years. I don't know much about his life apart from the fact that he became Chief Postmaster of Birmingham and was a dedicated union man. There are photographs of my grandparents with large groups of people at conferences. My grandfather's work ethic, once he retired, was channelled into the garden at their new home, and it was his absolute pride and joy while the house was my Nanna's domain.

As you looked down the garden from the kitchen window, there were specific areas. The gladioli in the bed in front of the window were usually salmon pink; there was the rose garden, with four beautifully manicured beds and a bird bath in the centre; a lush lawn; and four enormous conifer trees! When I was about six, I tried to learn to ride a bike and managed to cycle straight into one of the very unforgiving conifer trees. It was unscathed; I wasn't.

Beyond the conifers was an orchard, with Bramley apples, eating apples, plums, and pears. All of these fruits, and many others bought from the beautiful farm shops in the Vale of Evesham, would be lovingly prepared and bottled by Nanna and stored in a huge wooden dresser. The Bramley apples were wrapped up in newspaper, put in crates, and stored in the rafters of the garage for the winter months.

Beyond the orchard was the vegetable patch. It included an incredible array of canes for broad beans and runner beans, tomatoes which tasted incredible, lovely little potatoes, and many different greens! My Grandad spent most of his days in the garden and he liked things to look right. There was an incredibly long drive up to the bungalow with a high hedge, which he kept beautifully manicured; you would have struggled to see a leaf or branch out of place.

Now this all sounds idyllic, and in many ways it was. But there was a darker side to my stays. There was a little room at the back of the garage, a spare bedroom I suppose for guests, or maybe it could have been used as an office. For me, it signified a very unsafe space and a place of abuse. Abuse that made me feel ashamed, dirty, and left me with a nasty feeling about myself and who I was. This abuse wasn't dealt out by my grandparents, but by someone else. Someone I would face many, many years later! Those childhood experiences really changed how I viewed my body and ultimately tainted what I thought love was about. I tried on many different occasions to bring this nasty stuff to the attention of my parents, but I wasn't heard. I wasn't believed.

I can remember one particular situation when I found myself hiding in the rhododendron bushes in the grounds of the lovely school I attended, shaking uncontrollably with shame and fear about what had happened to me. I tried to explain, but yet again was silenced. The only acknowledgment I got was that I had said what I needed to say, and that it didn't need to be mentioned again! It was swept under the rug, a nasty secret not to be discussed. Those early experiences made me feel incredibly unsure of myself and started a very skewed view of my body, sex, and the opposite sex.

I was being silenced, and the message coming through loud and clear was that my voice did not matter. I did not deserve to be heard.

During my time at that school, my sister joined there. She had a bit of a reputation for being accident prone, and I can vividly remember playing netball and hearing a familiar scream! She had fallen and cracked her head open on a low wall next to the netball courts. I ran off the court in the middle of the game, scooped my sister up off the ground, and ran with her through the school and up a steep flight of stairs to the first aid room. That was an instinct that has never left me! If someone is in distress or injured, I need to help – it's what I do almost without thinking.

On that occasion, my sister was taken to hospital and had to have stitches in her head, along with a stern warning to go steady.

School just happened around me; there were no particular highs or lows. Then it was time for secondary school, which was about 15 miles from where we lived. I remember the daily journey as being high speed, sickness-inducing trips round very windy lanes. And there were many, many, many occasions when I arrived at school having thrown up on my way there or just as we arrived. There were a few reasons for this: my dad loved cars and speed; and we were usually running late. Not a great combination, and certainly not the best start to your day.

There were some amazing teachers who did their level best to create an enjoyable and engaging place to learn, and once I found subjects that I was good at, finally my report card started to look much brighter.

There were, though, some not-so-great experiences. We were expected to wear green capes in the winter months and had to walk into the town to the church and the library. We looked like a line of trees shuffling along and got some serious stick from kids at the high school. I also remember history lessons when the teacher would bring in her little Scotty dogs. They used to nip you on the back of your legs, so lessons were spent with your feet tucked under you as you sat precariously on your chair – not the best environment for concentration. My memories of this school are vivid and varied, but then everything changed.

When I was 12, my parents decided to move from the successful pub and all its regulars, to take on a different project. This might seem like a strange decision, but the brewery who owned the pub put the rent up due to its success, which changed the profitability for my parents. So, they bought a very old building in a pretty little village a few miles away, where my mum had grown up.

The building was an old pub that had previously been a workhouse, and from what I can remember it was made up of one slightly larger and two small cottages. My mum and dad managed to borrow money for the massive renovations that were required, bringing this project to fruition with blood, sweat, and tears, and many, many, many sleepless nights. My room was on the first floor on the front of the house and, as it was an incredibly old building, none of the floors upstairs were level.

I do have some happy memories of that place, but a lot of sad ones, as my parents' marriage ended when I was 13 and my sister was eight. We stayed with Mum, and she spent the next few years working incredible hours to keep a roof over our heads. The bailiffs visited and were sent away, and she just kept on. In all, she and, later, my sister ran the restaurant for 21 years with a small team, winning prestigious awards before Mum retired. The business took a toll on my mum's health at the same time as she faced personal challenges, including the loss of my grandmother. It was hard to watch the good times and then some very sad times.

When my parents went their separate ways, it was incredibly tough on me and my sister, but the other change was our schooling. We had to move from a very privileged, all girls' private school to the local mixed comprehensive. I wasn't comfortable around boys; I was scared of them.

When I have looked back at my school reports (found whilst moving house recently), it seems my confidence in my own abilities just plummeted after the move. From being enthusiastic and enjoying learning, I went to at times not wanting to take part at all! I went on to sit my 'O' levels and 'GCSE' exams, but my once expected 'A' in German came out as a GCSE grade 3! The marks weren't horrific across the board, but the additional nightmare of my dad's girlfriend dying during the main week of my exams didn't really help. I wasn't allowed to attend her funeral, and I wasn't allowed to support my dad either. I don't think he ever got over it. Years later, he asked me to find her grave and put flowers there.

By that stage at school, I just didn't want to focus on subjects that I felt I wasn't any good at. By contrast, my sister came away from the same school with amazing grades. It didn't help that I was on the receiving end of bullying; I just didn't feel comfortable or fit in, and certain people enjoyed pointing that out.

I have always enjoyed writing. When my parents used to argue, I can remember writing about it. But I wrote about little animal characters rather than humans; a family of little hedgehogs. I think I was trying to make sense of what was happening around me, and I couldn't. I look back now and remember my dad writing letters to Mum to try to explain how he felt, because every session of raised voices never brought a happy conclusion. Eventually, they concluded that parting was better all round.

As I neared the end of my time at school, I decided that I wanted to go to the local college instead of staying on for 'A' levels which, in my eyes, would only bring further humiliation.

I got my place at college and retook English Language, achieving a much more acceptable 'C'. I also enrolled on a full-time secretarial course, where I learned shorthand, typing, office practice, accounts, and a few other subjects. I loved my days at college, as there was a sense of freedom, and the tutors were great. Mrs Cadman, who taught me Accounts, left a lasting impression on me, and my grades reflected that. The bottom of my report for that year says, 'A conscientious student who is making good progress.' Now that's a bit more positive!

Initially, I had enrolled at college for two years, but at the end of the first year I decided I didn't want any more formal education, and I preferred to start work. This decision was not well received by my parents.

I wanted independence; I wanted to earn; I wanted to meet different people. That need to meet different people has been lifelong, because I find people fascinating. Yes, over the years I've met people who have made me feel incredibly inferior and useless, but thankfully, I've also met some incredible people in amazing places.

I think I have always been the odd one out in my family, and I didn't want to join the family business. I waited on tables for the big events like weddings (of which there were an amazing amount), Christmas, and New Year. But I didn't like being looked down on! I wanted to make my own way, and the first step towards that, and independence, was learning to drive at the age of 17. There was some transport from the village, but it was only one bus every hour. So, I learnt to drive, passing my test the first time – to the amazement of everyone around me!

Both my parents had a love of cars and driving, and I think they both owned beautiful sports cars at different points in their lives. I quite openly admit that I also love cars, and I am a bit of a car snob. I once dreamed of having a Lotus Elise! However, experiences later in my life made me review that, and I don't fancy being that close to the ground any more! My first car was actually a blue Mini, NOD915W. My dad originally had other ideas, and he took me to a local garage where there was a banana yellow Austin Allegro. (No thanks, Dad). My little blue Mini gave me the freedom I craved.

I did have a few hair-raising moments in the car, though. I was always happy to drive friends who didn't have their own wheels to parties, clubs, and on dates! On one occasion, a good friend of mine, who lived in the same little village, arranged for us to meet a lad and his friend on a double date. As it turned out, my trusted Mini got us to our destination, and we had a good night. We dropped off one passenger, and then it came to dropping off my friend's date. There was a trading estate and service road opposite where he lived. At some point before midnight, we parked up and all started chatting, and there was a bit of snogging in the back, with me curled up on the front seats. We all fell asleep, but were rudely awakened by the local police officer, as the windows were steamed up! Initially, I was incredibly scared and felt really stupid, but we all saw the funny side after he walked away!

There was another time when there were six people in my Mini. As visibility wasn't great, we all nearly snuffed it on a mini-island in a little village, because I just couldn't see out for all the heads and arms! My thoughts on road safety have since changed, but my Mini was my first taste of independence.

With the guiding hand of Mrs Cadman from college, I applied for a maternity leave post for six months with a building society. The only downside I could see was that they wanted someone with experience, but I needed to gain experience. After two interviews, I successfully got a job! Not the maternity cover, but a cashier's post that they then mentioned was available. It was my first proper job, and I was so delighted at starting work.

I loved meeting different people every day and getting to know all the regular customers. The owner of the local chip shop would bring his takings in, with the notes rolled up and smelling of the fish and chips. Challenge number one was rolling them out, in order to count the hundreds of pounds.

My grandmother had been a postmistress for many years in a tiny post office and shop, and I knew from stories my dad told me that she could add up column after column of numbers in her head. I didn't have that skill to the same degree, but numbers didn't worry me. So most of the time cashing up at the end of the day wasn't too much of a problem.

I worked with a lovely team and got to know people who worked for other financial institutions, like the bank over the way and the building society two doors down. I was really proud of myself that I had gained a job with prospects, and I learned quickly and started taking the formal exams which would enable me to progress. When I look back, I realise that I wanted to move up the ladder much quicker than was the norm.

Being in that branch brought about one huge change in my life that I could never have imagined. Back in the late 1980s, to open an account you had to fill in reams of forms and usually be invited in to talk to the Manager or a member of the team.

A lovely gentleman visited the branch to ask about a particular account and followed the process of making the appointment. It was suggested that I do the interview with him, and I found myself sitting across the table from a very attractive man, who was forthright but incredibly polite. Once he had completed the forms and left the branch, I had his complete credentials – age, marital status, occupation, etc.

Over the following few weeks, as the opening of his account was processed, I had to make a few telephone calls to him and to his lovely secretary. Once all of this had been completed, he arrived in the branch one day and I helped him with the transactions he needed. Then he asked me out! You could have knocked me over with a feather.

We arranged to go out at lunchtime the following Saturday. Now, I mentioned earlier that cashing up wasn't usually a problem for me – but it was on the day of that first date! We had had an incredibly busy morning in the branch, and I was quite nervous about my upcoming date – not a great combination. I openly admit that I was incredibly naive about dating and the opposite sex. But he waited patiently until we had finally cashed up, and then took me out for a drink in a pub that would become our regular haunt. I absolutely fell for him, hook, line, and sinker!

From the paperwork he had completed for his account, I already knew that Stan was 16 years older than me, was widowed, had a young daughter, that he worked in a job that meant he travelled a lot, and lots more besides. Stan was born in Delhi in India and came to Stourbridge at the age of nine, with his parents, brothers, and sister. His youngest sister was born in the UK. Stan had gone to the local comprehensive then gained a place at the local Boys' Grammar School – the first pupil of colour.

I find this hard to write about, because the person I met was just Stan. I didn't care about the colour of his skin, or his religion. I just fell in love. Over the years that followed, we partied hard, but we were made to feel very uncomfortable about our relationship by some and welcomed with open arms by others. As time went on, I started to become more involved in his family life and spent time with his daughter Sarah, which involved some funny moments.

I went round to the house after work one day and offered to bath Sarah, which was not something she particularly enjoyed. I managed it, though, and afterwards wrapped her in a big towel and proceeded to try and put her in her pyjamas. Part of her bathing ritual was talcum powder. I was still wearing my pale blue uniform for work, and suddenly Sarah grabbed the talcum powder and squeezed it. Choking, we both ended up in a cloud of Johnson's baby powder. My suit never looked quite the same again, but we were both laughing!

I soon realised that I was walking into a different way of life, but one that most of the time I felt able to enjoy. However, as time went on, family pressures from both sides took its toll on us and our relationship, and after two years together, we parted company and went our separate ways. It was not something either of us wanted really, but we just didn't seem to be able to overcome the difficulties and input from other people. In those first few years, though, I had learnt what love was and what being in a relationship was all about – love, care, and give and take.

There were a few occasions when I thought things would turn out differently. My mum arranged a very lavish party for my 21st birthday at the restaurant, but Stan had decided he wanted to take me to Paris for the occasion, so there was a bit of a clash. In the end, we went to Paris for four days, arriving back home on the afternoon of the party.

Unfortunately, the trip had not really gone the way I thought it would. We got to the top of the Eiffel Tower, and I had anticipated Stan getting down on one knee to propose to me. But no! We just walked back down. We returned to England on the ferry, but I've never been great on the water since my dad nearly drowned us whilst out on a speed boat in Tenby.

When Stan and I got on the ferry, everything was tied down. Everything! It was so choppy you couldn't walk around, although that definitely wasn't something I felt able to do anyway, as I was too busy throwing up. Eventually, I arrived at my mum's restaurant looking a lovely shade of green, and just about made it through my birthday party!

I think it would be fair to say that Stan and I both went off the rails a bit after we separated. I had been shown love, and I tried to find that elsewhere without success. I now realise that I just gave my body away to others without a thought of the impact that would have on me, and this is definitely something I regret. One night, I went to a party at a big hotel in Birmingham with a friend of mine. I met a guy the same age as me, who seemed nice, and we got on well. He was only visiting the city, as he lived down South, but we arranged to meet up. And over the following few months, I drove down to see him, and he drove up to see me.

He told me he was emigrating to Australia... and I told him I was pregnant. The two didn't match up! So, I made one of the toughest decisions of my life and had an abortion. All I will say on this is that I have carried guilt and shame ever since, but I made the only decision I could in the circumstances. I didn't tell anyone, except two friends who supported me, and I couldn't tell my mum. Years later, I was forced to tell her, and I think it shocked her to the core.

Work became my focus, and I went to work at another building society, and moved into my first flat to be near to work. The flat was in a city, and the road I lived on was on the edge of an area made up of a huge diversity of nationalities, cultures, and faiths.

Moving out from home, though, caused more fallings out, and I didn't leave in a flurry of help and blessings. All I had was a second-hand cooker, kindly donated by someone I worked with, and my grandmother's old brown, two-seater sofa with wooden arms. Everything seemed to be brown: brown carpets, brown curtains, and brown sofa.

My two major purchases were a new bed and a washing machine, but the machine caused a fall-out with my neighbours beneath me. My dad had offered to help and plumb in the machine, but the only problem was he hadn't tightened the connections properly. So I met my new neighbours when water started pouring through their ceiling!

Now I had my independence, I needed to keep the roof over my head. I got a staff mortgage, which was quite the norm back then, but it still meant I had very little spare money. To boost my funds, I got myself a part-time job in a beautiful little country pub; I knew how to pull a pint, and I liked meeting people. For a while, my life revolved around work.

I am sure you have certain foods that you remember from your childhood or a period in your adult life. In my case, I survived many weeks on a diet of beans on toast, or sardines on toast, as I never quite got round to stopping long enough to cook a proper meal.

I liked my building society job, but it was at a time when you worked with brokers who would introduce business. I remember a very lovely Asian gentleman who provided lots of good applications. My boss at the time very unceremoniously advised me that I could deal with him, as I knew what *they* were like! I will leave that thought with you.

I dealt with the new applications and the repossessions, which wasn't fun, and I worked crazy hours trying to prove my worth. For years I kept a letter from a gentleman I helped, who was relocating with his company. It was a letter of appreciation for my determination to get his mortgage sorted quickly so that he could move within a very quick timescale. But I just wanted to help whoever I could; I didn't care about the colour of their skin or nationality! My boss at the time, however, had a very different view.

On one occasion, I found myself in the little interview room with a knife being held at my throat, because the customer on the other side of the desk didn't think I was taking him seriously. Thank goodness for the panic button under the desk!

On another night, I had been working very late in the office on my own – probably not the best plan; if I recall correctly, it was a Tuesday evening. So, I finally decided it was time to go home, made my way out of the office and locked up. The building was on one of the city's usually fairly quiet roads, but not that night. I suddenly found myself facing a line of mounted police, with an enormous crowd of football fans behind them. I very quickly went back inside and patiently waited until they had all passed by.

Situations like these didn't help the stress levels I was already under, and my boss decided I couldn't cope, so I was pushed out. I think he enjoyed that process.

I moved away from the city and bought myself a little, new-build house. My dad had been around when I moved, and he offered to help again, this time with putting shelves up! Don't get me wrong, my dad created amazing things with his lathe, and I still have beautiful bowls he made. However, he suggested creating a little group of shelves by the front door in between the little kitchen and lounge. It was all open plan – compact and bijou, some might say. So, he got the wood, marked out where the shelves would go, and started drilling. Within a couple of seconds, a jet of water was shooting out of the wall, across the room, and hitting the wall on the other side! Until that point, I had never realised the power of water under pressure. Cue a scramble for the stopcock, and then mopping up!

Part of my move involved rebuilding my relationship with my mum, but her first visit to my new home didn't go quite according to plan either. I had invited her and my stepdad John over for Sunday lunch. My mum was an amazing cook, so I was already a bit nervous about making a nice meal for the three of us. They arrived, and all seemed well until my mum started with a nosebleed. This wasn't unusual for her, but this time there was no stopping it! So, our quiet Sunday dinner turned into hours at the local hospital.

I joined a temping agency and worked for all sorts of companies, some for just a few days or weeks, but I learnt a lot in that time! Then I was sent for an interview with a telecommunications company who wanted an admin assistant, tea maker, and general dogsbody. I started as a temp there, and then was offered a permanent job.

My role was to help create some organisation with installations, dealing with BT and the engineers. And I absolutely loved it, as no two days were the same. Then as things started to get busier and more organised, they needed someone on site to train the customers on how to use the new systems. When another admin assistant joined the company, I moved out of the office and did the onsite training visits.

We had customers who had multiple sites throughout the country, and the staff at each site had to be trained in the same way. One week I would be in Scotland, the next in Wales or the south coast. I loved the variety, along with the banter with the customers and the engineers. The only bit I wasn't keen on was someone else planning my diary – or should I say, not planning.

One day, I needed to be onsite in Poole in Dorset at 7am for a big customer and make a site visit in Warwick on the way back to the office. I gained a speeding ticket on the way down to site and on the way back up!

I remember cold calling at a foundry in the Black Country and asking if they needed a new telephone system. They did, as they were renovating the offices that hadn't changed in over 50 years. So, I ended up trailing through their factory to carry out an initial site survey. A foundry is a manufacturing factory that produces castings by melting metal, pouring the molten liquid into a mould, and then solidifying it. They are incredibly hot and dirty environments – that's just how it is.

The next time I went through the foundry to carry out a much more detailed survey, I made sure I was more suitably dressed for the conditions. However, when the work was done and I turned up to do the training dressed in clothes more suited to the foundry, the staff were all sitting in their beautiful new offices, dressed in suits! Not my finest hour.

The biggest site I worked on was owned by a huge American firm, and the installation took months. When it came to the training schedule for about 150 staff, we had it all planned out and it was undertaken in small groups throughout the site. I loved that part of the job!

They had a head receptionist who sat in the most amazing reception area. My boss at the time informed me that I must turn up in my best clothes, as I would be in the main reception for the receptionist's full day training. I did as I was told and turned up in a mauve culotte suit and white shirt (very much the fashion of the day!). But there was work going on to redo the ceiling, so the head receptionist and I spent the entire day with bits dropping on us, covering us in plaster dust, paint, and stray bits from the ceiling. I handed my boss the dry-cleaning bill for my clothes and decided from then on that I would decide what I wore to work.

One of the greatest parts of that job was going on site, usually being greeted by someone very irate and swearing, because things didn't always go to plan with the installations or tying up with the local exchange. I would sit with a blank sheet of paper and let the person rant about what wasn't right or what needed fixing, then I would go away and, nine times out of ten, by close of business all items on that list had been resolved by me or with the help of one of the engineers on site. There was always a sense of getting the job done and usually having a good laugh at the same time.

I was onsite once at a huge warehouse which had had a new phone system and public address system installed. Sadly, I had to test the public address system for the first time, to ask for the building to be evacuated because someone had been crushed under a forklift truck. I even heard my dulcet tones over the PA system at a couple of football clubs! I had gained some confidence in this job, though, and didn't mind if people heard my voice. And I have a smile on my face as I remember these times.

After a while, a competitor approached me to join them to do sales and training, and I was ready for a change. When I handed in my resignation, it was not a decision that my boss took well, locking me in an office so that I couldn't take my files, index cards, and customer details with me. Unnecessary, I feel.

When I moved, I worked out of a small office with a lady who wouldn't mind me saying she was larger than life in every sense. She was an amazing saleswoman with a real gift of the gab. It was only a small company, but they had many prestigious companies as their customers. One thing I didn't like doing wherever I worked, though, was cold calling, and I still don't much enjoy it now!

She handed me a business directory and said we needed to drum up some new business, then gave me a rough script to work from. But when I started at A, I very quickly realised that someone had already done that, so I went to Z and worked my way backwards. I cold called an advertising agency in the middle of Birmingham and asked my list of questions, and they did need my help. Hooray! An appointment was arranged for me to visit them in person.

I arrived a few days later and sat in the reception area of their very posh offices, looking at trade magazines. I opened one, and it was a full page spread of the agency and a local brewery. And there were quite a few faces I recognised! I was then ushered into the boardroom, where there were more framed photographs of people I knew.

We had the meeting, and the person I was chatting with said he thought he recognised me. He was right; I was the ex-girlfriend of one of his clients. When our meeting concluded, as I left I said, 'If you speak to Stan Fernandez, please send him my regards.' Yes, that's right, their client was my first love Stan who I hadn't seen for many years. I'd never stopped loving him, though, and I'd immediately spotted him amongst the photos on the boardroom wall.

I didn't think any more of it other than what an incredibly small world we live in! But later that same week, I was minding my own business sitting in the office I shared, when I heard a phone call come through downstairs. I could only hear, 'Yes, she works here. Yes, I can put you through.' When my phone rang and I answered it, the voice said, 'How are you?' I immediately turned white; the colour just drained from my face. In fact, the lady sitting across the desk thought someone had died, or something similar! As our conversation continued, the colour slowly returned to my face. So I pushed a note across the desk to reassure her, with one simple word: 'Stan!'.

We agreed to meet at the same pub that we used to go to, and at first we both stood very stiffly at an angle to each other at the bar. I don't think either of us knew what to do or what to say, but slowly we opened up to each other and shared some of what had happened since we'd separated. We both knew how we had felt about each other, but the outside pressures of family and work had been allowed to destroy how we truly felt.

Within a few weeks, some of our close family were made aware that we were back in touch, and within a few months a wedding was planned. We stood strong in our wish to be together, and our love story continued…

Chapter: Two

We got married in the same church in which my mother married, where I had been christened, and where numerous members of previous generations had been buried in the churchyard. It's a beautiful little church.

At this point, a bit of religious negotiation had to be undertaken. I grew up going to a Church of England church and schools that followed the same direction. Stan, however, was Catholic, and his faith meant a great deal to him. It turned out that the parish priest and the vicar had trained together at some point, so they decided they would share the service, and we couldn't have asked for anything better at that point in 1994. The photos of our wedding were beautiful and absolutely capture our love for each other.

In the months before the wedding, we had moved house, and the company Stan worked for approached him about a few overseas jobs. The one that caught his attention and then came to fruition was to be based in Mumbai (Bombay) for three years. His task involved the planning and opening of over one hundred ice cream stores and overseeing the ice cream factory that would supply them. As Stan was incredibly hardworking and highly respected, this was the next step in his career, and we would be joining him for this next stage.

There is a song with the words 'life is a rollercoaster', and certainly my married life has been referred to like that a few times.

Stan, Sarah, and I made an initial visit to Bombay to look around. We were flown Business Class, arriving in the middle of the night, which meant we didn't see the sprawling slums. But we were treated like royalty and the visit was mind-blowing.

I can remember a conversation that Stan and I had had much earlier in our relationship, about wanting to understand the country where he had been born and its culture. I got to see it, smell it, and experience it for myself, and although at times it was tough, I will never forget those times and experiences.

After our initial trip, we made the decision to embark on this adventure, and a big leaving party was arranged, and our belongings packed. The company Stan had been working with gave him a few gifts for the next chapter of his varied career, including three heavy duty trunks and a slightly smaller case. The smaller case became our medicine cabinet and was packed with malaria tablets, painkillers, Calpol, bandages, insect spray, dressings, plasters; the list was endless. We had our vaccinations and then, before we knew it, it was September, and we were flying off to start a new life. The three of us – Stan, Sarah, and me – and our worldly belongings were set up in two adjoining rooms in a hotel in Bombay.

I'm not sure I can find the words to explain the feeling of bombardment that you feel in a new place, a new way of life, a new culture. And also, Bombay never sleeps. The other overwhelming feeling I had was of shock at the immense wealth visible right next to a fishing village where the only belongings the fisherman and his family had were the sticks that held a sheet for them to sleep under and a cooking pot. We travelled past that fishing village every day for months on the way to Sarah's school.

New routines soon fell into place. Work for Stan was sometimes in Bombay, sometimes Puna, sometimes Delhi, sometimes much further away from Sarah and me.

School for Sarah, now ten years old, was the American School – a tiny school for expatriates, with teachers and staff of many different nationalities. Each day we would get in a taxi and travel to school, after having breakfast in the hotel restaurant or ordering room service.

Sarah had left a kind, loving, caring school in the UK, where she had excelled, and in many ways that made the new school and environment even harder for her to get used to. But, bless her, she got on with it, even with the bullying. Every morning, I would take Sarah into school and then head back to the only place I knew – our hotel.

After a couple of weeks, I got chatting to the school secretary who was Indian and married to an English guy. She asked what I was doing to fill my time, but I didn't really know. She explained that they were looking for a part-time secretary and asked if I would be interested. I didn't need asking twice! I was interviewed and got the job.

There was another lady in the office in charge of the finances; another Indian lady with an English husband. What an experience that was for me. Not only did I learn about the school and the budgets, but I learned so, so much more about culture and traditions.

We had the opportunity to go to the store openings – usually very lavish affairs at which the business was blessed, everyone was dressed beautifully, and a good time was had by all. We were also invited to weddings, festivals, and all sorts of different gatherings. And for each new gathering, I had to have a new saree.

Now, there is an art to putting on a saree, and it was a knack I didn't have, so a lovely lady from the hotel staff would come and help me to get dressed. I had incredibly beautiful sarees, and it was decided that the best way to make it easy for me to wear them was to have them stitched in a certain way so that I could just wrap them round me and keep them in place with various clips or poppers. I felt amazing in such beautiful clothes. There were some funny experiences along the way, as well as a few heart-stopping moments.

We tried to settle into a routine, but Sarah really wasn't a great fan of the local food. After a while, we found a little café called Under the Over, which was literally tucked under the main overpass through Bombay. That place, at least, provided food that we could both enjoy.

Lots of people talk about Delhi belly and getting used to the local food, with guidance to eat vegetarian food over meat, if possible. Well, we tried our best, but had a few bouts of upset stomachs and feeling under the weather. The food situation was improved, though, by invitations to the homes of other expatriates, who would wash absolutely everything they ate in Milton tablets to kill off as many germs as possible. We were also directed to a black-market shop that sold food items more appreciated by the expats. Cheddar cheese was high on the list, and I won't name the brands, but we needed soap, chocolate, water biscuits, tins of soup, and other very British items that were not readily available! Strangely, you could buy Cadbury's chocolate produced in India, but it tasted completely different. So probably once a week, we would go to this shop and come away with our little stash of items to be put in the tiny fridges in our hotel rooms.

A few weeks into working at the school, I started feeling below par but just put it down to the move, the heat, and the many changes that had occurred since we'd moved. There was a lovely Australian nurse who was part of the staff at the school and who kept an eye on the pupils and the staff. I went to her one day complaining of nausea and generally feeling very out of sorts. We had joked before this about our medicine case, and on this occasion, she very gently asked if there was a pregnancy test amongst the stash. I had to respond that I didn't know.

Later that day, I checked, and there wasn't, so I got one from the chemist. That lovely nurse had already sussed it, but I hadn't. So, the next thing I knew was that the test was positive, and we were calling home to let the family know that I was pregnant! We were absolutely thrilled! This was well received by some but, let's be honest, not by others.

Over the coming weeks, I went to appointments with an amazing gynaecologist. I used to travel to his office in a black and yellow taxi that you see in photographs and film footage of India. Travelling from the hotel, part of the journey was along Pedder Road, which is a busy main road with many sets of traffic lights. At each set, a tiny face would be pushed against the window, another little face begging. These children had limbs missing, horrendous scars, and were filthy; it's almost impossible to put into words. There I was, carrying a little baby who was having the best help and the best care, and those children pretty much had nothing!!

Stan worked incredibly long hours, but one of various situations we needed to resolve at that stage was our living accommodation. When we had first arrived in Bombay, the plan had been for a short stay in a hotel and then we would find and move into an apartment. But the cost of renting property was among the highest in the world at that point.

Our search began, and we looked at marble-floored apartments to rent near to Sarah's school, which the company had agreed to pay for. What no-one had bargained on was the fact that Stan had been born in India and, although he had a British passport and had lived almost all of his life in England, he was not someone the landlords wanted to rent to. If he had taken up Indian citizenship, they would not have been able to remove him from the property.

Discussions began: could it be rented to me? No! Could the company rent it? No! The upshot was we couldn't rent anywhere, so Plan B came into play. We moved from our original hotel into one of the most prestigious hotels in Bombay, and we set up home there. We needed a change of scenery from the two rooms in the original hotel, but this time we were all in one room. We absolutely made the best of it, though, and I have some great memories of the place, the staff, and the food. I have an image in my head now of getting dressed for a wedding, with Sarah, Stan, and I dressed in beautiful traditional clothes. We took so many photos in the room and in the foyer of the hotel.

I only have one saree I remember as not being so great; it was green and gold. I really struggled with morning sickness (and evening sickness) when I was pregnant, and I used to turn a strange green shade, so in one photograph it's difficult to distinguish me from the saree!

During my pregnancy I did have one particularly bad patch, when I got food poisoning. Not ideal! The company had arranged that we would have a car and driver who would take Stan where he needed to go, but also Sarah and me.

Our driver was the kindest, most gentle man, and he would be there waiting every morning in the little red car, and off we would go. On one particular day, we had taken Sarah to school, gone back to the hotel, and then I planned to go shopping. Kundan collected me as usual, but we had only travelled about a mile when I felt incredibly sick – to the point of asking him to stop so I could get out of the car and throw up! It's not something you want to be seen doing or happening to you in broad daylight in 40-degree temperatures.

Kundan took me straight back to my hotel, where I went to my room to lie down. Little did I know that Kundan had then gone to Stan's office, walked into a meeting, which could have got him sacked, and informed Stan that 'Madam is sick'. I found out afterwards that Kundan had been widowed and he didn't want anything to happen to 'Madam'. I spent three days lying flat in bed on doctors' orders if I wanted to keep my baby! It was incredibly scary, only moving to throw up or go to the toilet.

The months rolled on, and Sarah was a little more settled in school but definitely not enjoying it. Another highlight was when the Plague was declared in a neighbouring state, so they had to disinfect the school and classrooms. DDT was used – a substance long banned in the UK. You are meant to leave the building empty after spraying it, but within a few hours staff and pupils were back at their desks.

In the February – specifically the 14th of February, 1995 – I decided to surprise Stan at his office. I had arranged to have a head massage and my hair done in the salon in the hotel, as I wanted to look as glamorous as the beautiful women I saw around me every day. I put on a heavy patterned, pink and gold bodice, with a plain shocking pink saree. I think at this point my body was getting used to being pregnant, and I was too. So, I got all dressed up in my finery and got a taxi to his office. Stan was absolutely blown away that I wanted to make such an effort, and his staff were so, so kind and complimentary. Work stopped, and we went out to lunch. I'm not known for being spontaneous, but I absolutely loved every minute of that special day.

I continued my weekly visits to the gynaecologist, and then it was time for us to decide where our little one was going to be born. There was a local private maternity hospital, and a visit had been arranged for another expat lady who was due around the same time, so we decided to go together.

I had only had experience of being in hospital back in the UK a couple of time, although lots of times visiting relatives. But this was a very different experience. It was an old building, and it was incredibly hot. We were shown the theatre and delivery room, the area where the babies were being bathed – two or three through the same water – and then the nursery where the babies were sleeping. I asked why there were nets over the cot. Answer: to keep the cockroaches out!

I will be really honest and say that up until that point I had been going with the 'I'm happy to have my baby in Bombay'. But not after that visit. I rang Stan when I got back to the hotel and said he could book a flight for me and Sarah for whenever he thought was best, and I would have our baby in the UK. As it turned out, it's a good job he did, because at the time when Georgina would have been born there, the hospital was closed due to a legionella.

Plans were then made for our return to the UK, but we would be leaving Stan in India to continue with his job. That time was hard on all of us. Sarah and I were booked on a Business Class flight back to the UK, but I felt very torn about the decision to head home. I'd already faced a difficult dilemma in the January when my grandmother died, as I had wanted to be at her funeral but knew I could only fly back once before our baby was born. I adored my grandmother, but didn't travel back for her funeral. So now we were leaving Bombay, without Stan, and not knowing when we would be back. Sarah and I were going to be staying with Stan's parents in their home, and would be near other family.

Bombay airport is a crazy place. We had loads of luggage and hand luggage, so we went through the process of checking in our bags and then going to security checks. I have never felt so humiliated by another woman as I was that day. I was seven months' pregnant and wearing quite traditional Indian clothes – a shalwar chemise. The trousers had a drawstring waist, which was perfect for an ever-changing waistline.

The humiliation was inflicted upon me by a female security guard. She poked me literally from head to toe in places you shouldn't be poked, whilst Sarah just stood about ten feet away, looking scared and confused by what was happening. Eventually the guard let me go, but I walked away feeling dirty and distressed. That walk suddenly turned into a run as the flight was boarding, and it was a long way to the gate and to the plane.

We finally made it, only to be greeted by an air stewardess who barked orders at us to get to our seats. I am sure that my choice of traditional dress hadn't done me any favours that day. I don't think the guard liked the fact I was a white woman in traditional dress, and sadly I don't think the neatly dressed stewardess approved either, and she continued with her gruff manner until we had taken off.

I was in a great deal of abdominal pain, but just gritted my teeth and held tight to Sarah. About half an hour later, I got up to speak to the stewardess and to ask if they had any passengers who had been highlighted as needing help or special assistance. I knew the travel agent had mentioned about my pregnancy, as I was flying back at the last possible stage.

The stewardess said, 'No.' But I gently but firmly informed her that I was pregnant, even if I didn't look it! I also said that the travel agent had informed the airline of my condition, and that her assistance would have been more helpful rather than her barking at me! She apologised, and about an hour later a very expensive bottle of champagne was handed to me by way of a gift to celebrate the new arrival!

I have never been more relieved to arrive back in the UK than I was that day. I had lost a lot of weight rather than gained it whilst I was pregnant, due to a nasty combination of morning sickness, food poisoning, and stress. The consultant in Bombay had made it very clear that I would need to go for blood tests and be looked after once I was back home.

I have to say that I smile every time I think of the first appointment at the local maternity hospital in the UK. My doctor had arranged for me to see a gynaecologist, and to have a scan and blood tests. When I arrived in the waiting area, I overheard a conversation between the receptionists. They were looking at a set of patient notes and were concerned that they had a lady from India who had an appointment, but no translator had been arranged. They sounded genuinely concerned.

On the off-chance it was me they were discussing, I went to the desk and very politely explained that I might have a foreign surname and had arrived from India, but I wouldn't need a translator and that I could speak the language! The look of relief, and then the laughter at the situation, made that first visit a whole lot easier. Sadly, I got quite used to going for scans and blood tests, but they kept an amazing eye on me throughout! My consultant advised me that although I wasn't in the best of health, he was sure my baby was!

I started with contractions, or what I thought were contractions, on the Saturday, so I was dropped off at hospital by my dad. He was the nearest person who could drive at the time, as I was living with Stan's parents in their home.

Stan was contacted in India so that he could get a flight home, but that didn't quite go according to plan! A fleet of new planes, which had been delivered to a well-known airline, were facing technical issues so there were no flights leaving Bombay!

Jayne – Aunty Jam, as she was affectionally known by Georgina – stepped forward as my birthing helper, and our daughter finally arrived on Sunday afternoon. Jayne was the first person to see Georgina, and that bond is still strong some 27 years later.

Whilst still in India, Stan, Sarah, and I had discussed names, and we had decided on Georgina for a girl and George for a boy. George was also a previous family name on Stan's side of the family. And when Georgina then arrived on St George's Day, we knew we had chosen the right name.

I managed to speak to Stan on the phone after the birth, but was desperate for him to get home. When he arrived on the Tuesday, he came straight to the hospital, and the nurses at the maternity hospital were amazing. I was in a six-bedded ward, but when they heard Stan had made it back and would be visiting that day, they set aside a separate room so we could be together. I was so, so grateful for this.

Sarah came to visit us in hospital and was introduced to her little sister. I will be honest and say I suddenly felt completely overwhelmed by doubts of whether I could cope with a new baby. Of course I did manage, but I didn't find it easy, and my own health wasn't great for some time. When Georgina was christened, I looked a shadow of my former self. The pictures of that day were never on display.

We soon got into the habit of being together as a family, and slowly but surely things became more settled. We decided that we would have our own house back, as we had rented it out when we left for India. But that was not as easy as we had hoped, and the gentleman in it didn't appreciate the urgency. So I ended up helping him to find somewhere else to live, in order that he would vacate our house! It was an extra stress I didn't need.

Our family of four had some serious decisions to make, too. Were we going back to India? Stan didn't really have an option; it was a three-year contract. However, the education wasn't working well for Sarah, and having a new-born baby and living in hotels didn't seem a good option, as there was still no resolution with the housing situation.

After a lot of discussion, an alternative plan was formulated. We would move to Dubai, where there were better schools and better housing, and Stan could travel easily back and forth to India. On paper, that looked like a grand plan, and some of it did work. All our belongings were packed up again, and another adventure began in January 1996. However, the red tape in arranging this move proved to be unbelievable. We needed a company to sponsor us, and that was found. Schooling – a primary school was recommended, and forms completed; then finding a home – we didn't want to be living in hotel rooms any more.

The only thing that stopped these plans going smoothly was when I became ill when Georgina was just six months old. I was experiencing horrendous stomach cramps and was struggling to function. I made an appointment at the doctors, which was a short walk from home, but I got as far the reception desk, gave my name, and then collapsed in the waiting room.

Every time I hear an ambulance siren, I remember how grateful I am for the speed at which the ambulance came for me on that day. I was taken to the local hospital, where I underwent various tests and observations. The verdict was that I had a strangulated colon and required emergency surgery, so off I went to the operating theatre. I remember very little of this experience, apart from my overwhelming fear of whether I would be ok. Thankfully, during this visit to the doctors, Georgina was with her grandparents, and they were taking great care of her whilst the medics looked after me.

Sarah had already started school, so she had to return to Dubai as an unaccompanied minor, which meant travelling on the flight back in the care of one of the stewardesses at all times, then being met by a dear friend in Dubai. As a family, we had got used to getting on and off planes and navigating our way through airports, but I missed Sarah so much during this time and felt very guilty that we couldn't all be together.

I stayed with Stan's brother Tony and his partner Jayne (Aunty Jam) when I came out of hospital, as the surgery meant that I couldn't carry anything. The hardest part was that included lifting Georgina. I will always be grateful for the love and support I received throughout this tough time, and it was so hard on all of us – Sarah and Stan in Dubai, and Georgina and me in Worcester.

Chapter: Three

So back to our life in Dubai. In the 1960s, groups of bungalows were built as temporary housing for the oil workers. These buildings were only supposed to be there for about five to ten years, but they remained and became little mini housing villages for expats. One of these bungalows became our home, with a mixture of our furniture and belongings from England and large amounts of IKEA items to fill in where needed.

I have such beautiful memories of Dubai. We created a beautiful home and we settled into the routines of school and nursery, while Stan continued to travel and work in India.

On my first visit to the school that Sarah attended, I met a lovely lady called Catharine, who would become a very dear friend and my rock when things didn't quite go to plan. This included supporting us when Georgina was rushed into hospital one night with a raging temperature, delirious, and unresponsive! We travelled in a taxi to the American Hospital, and when the driver realised I had a sick child, we almost flew there, Sarah and I cradling Georgina in the back of the taxi.

After three days of amazing care, Georgina was on the mend. One of the amazing nurses had to put a cannula in Georgina's hand, but in order to make it less scary, she put cream on to numb the area, then a plaster for her to draw on. She put one on each of Georgina's hands and drew faces so they could talk to each other while the numbing worked, then she put the needle in without Georgina even flinching.

Georgina has always liked food, but trying to persuade her to eat when she was in hospital wasn't easy. One of the nurses suggested ordering takeaway pizza that they would deliver to the hospital, and even now we joke that the olives on the takeaway pizza helped her to get better. Maybe that's why Georgina still has a love of olives!

Dubai had a huge expat community, but most social events were geared to families, and for quite a lot of the time I would have the girls while Stan would be travelling. It had been decided that if he worked in India for six weeks at a time, and then came home to spend a little time with us, it would be more cost effective than bobbing back and forth. We looked forward so much to his return, which was usually for a week, and then off he went again. In his absence, having a group of friends who also had small children became my lifeline and sanity, with picnics in the park and playdays at each other's homes.

We had family come out to visit for birthdays and Christmas, which was amazing, and we also had unexpected distant family visit, as well as work colleagues of Stan's. The 'tennis ball curry' episode was when a cousin of Stan's visited from Kuala Lumpur, and I felt I had to impress on the food front. I made a meatball curry, which Stan's mum had shown me how to cook. You are meant to have small meatballs, probably 3cm maximum in diameter, which are filled with spices and then cooked in a rich sauce. However, I didn't quite get the meatball size right, and they were like tennis balls. It still causes a smile when I make this dish, but my meatballs are definitely the right size now!

One visitor was a lovely Canadian gentleman who was a colleague of Stan's and who spent a couple of days with us. His visit really helped me, because he was so kind and generous with his words of support for me being in a foreign country with a different culture. That really meant a lot. Some of our family, on both sides, had been against the move to Dubai, but I think over time we showed them that we could cope and actually thrive in a different place.

Stan worked incredibly long hours, and when he did make it back to Dubai, we would try to plan some proper rest and recuperation. We enjoyed a few trips to Oman, and there was an oasis called Hatta which we drove to. One of our trips to Hatta didn't quite go to plan, though, and we ended up lost in the wadi (riverbed), literally sitting in our Land Rover with the girls in the back, praying that we would be safe overnight and that it wouldn't rain and wash us away. To explain, this was back around 1997, with no sophisticated satnav to help us navigate where we were, and we found ourselves in the middle of nowhere in the middle of the night. We weren't driving on our equivalent in the UK of B roads; there *weren't* any roads!

As a family, we did the tourist bits as well, like the 4x4 trips over the sand dunes and visited the Dubai Museum. I loved to go to the souks to buy spices and clothes, and there were different districts with more specific shops. Stan's mum loved to sew, and she made her own clothes as well as clothes for family members and even bridesmaids' dresses, so she loved visiting all the fabric shops. Each time she went home, her case was full of fabric, and we would take even more back for her when we came back. She also had a favourite place to buy shoes and sandals, and many years later she could still be seen wearing one of her favourite pairs of sandals.

The spice markets were incredible, with all the vibrant colours and smells. Another much visited area in Dubai is the gold souk, where hundreds of shops of all sizes sell every item of gold jewellery you could possibly think of. This includes incredibly traditional pieces, wedding items, modern designs, and some would make whatever item you wanted. It's hard to describe it, and particularly difficult to explain how the wealth exuded from that place. But Dubai, when we were lucky enough to live there, was a great place to be as an expat.

We also got the chance to travel back to Mumbai (Bombay) after Georgina was born, and we made a trip to Nepal, flying into the smog-covered city of Kathmandu. We trekked with

Sarah and Georgina and went to the Buddhist temples high in the mountains above Kathmandu. Georgina was carried in a metal-framed carrier on our backs. We had a driver, who was our guide on that trip, and he knew all the best places to stop for amazing food. We stayed in the most incredible places, and watched the sunrise from a hut in the Annapurna range of mountains. We also visited the spectacular Pokhara lakes. As I am recalling all of this, I have a huge smile on my face, as it was such an incredibly special trip.

The return journey to Dubai didn't quite go according to plan, though. You needed to obtain a visa to enter India to travel on to Nepal, where you needed another visa. I was tasked with sorting out all the paperwork at the Indian consulate in Dubai, but I didn't quite get it right. I got the visas for Nepal right, but not for India. I had got a visa, but it was a single-entry visa not multi-entry! So, we travelled to Bombay and then on to Nepal with no problems. The return trip saw us arrive in Bombay airport, tired and bedraggled, and looking forward to seeing friends and staying back in Bombay for a few days. We got to passport control, showed our paperwork, and were then informed we couldn't come into the country as we didn't have the necessary visa. I wanted the ground to swallow me up!

We spent five hours sitting on the floor of the sweltering airport, trying to contact people who could help us resolve this dreadful situation. Sarah was 12 at the time, and Georgina was just two. It was finally resolved by one of the very wealthy sponsors of the company Stan worked with in India. I would absolutely love to go back to Nepal, but I learnt from that experience to always check, check, and triple check documents for travel!

I mentioned earlier that at school I loved to swim, and the complex we lived on in Dubai had the benefit of a huge pool and restaurant, as well as access to the beach and the sea. This was amazing for all of us, as Sarah also loved to swim, and Georgina literally took to it like a duck to water!

Our life there probably sounds picture perfect, but it wasn't always like that. One of the hardest times was when Stan arrived on a plane from Bombay on one occasion and didn't know where he was or, at one point, who he was. This situation frightened all of us. Stan wasn't a fan of hospitals for all sorts of different reasons, and just felt he would get better, but he had been unable to work for a couple of weeks, which was absolutely unheard of. You could have been forgiven for thinking that maybe he'd had too much to drink on the flight home, but that wasn't what he did. And we were unable to find out what had happened in the few days before he became so poorly.

We were due to travel back to the UK on one of our visits paid for by the company, but Stan's ill health was a real concern, so the company decided that when we got there, all four of us would visit the tropical diseases institute in London. We wanted to try to ascertain what had been wrong with Stan and Georgina, and also to check Sarah and me over. Many discussions, many tests, and trips to London, still didn't provide us with any answers, and we returned to Dubai somewhat reassured that there was nothing wrong with us that we could put a name to. As I look back now, there were other times when Stan was ill which he just shrugged off as unimportant. To be honest, I don't think he ever regained a clean bill of health.

We spent three years in Dubai, and in the last few months there were lots of discussions as to where we would be going next. Stan made a visit to Moscow, as there was potentially a position available there, but it was around the time when there were kidnappings and shootings of the expat community. Stan was guarded the whole time he was there, and it was explained that this would have to be the case for the whole family. He decided it was not a place he wanted to take us, nor a way he wanted to live. In the end, we decided that we would head back to the UK and see what happened next.

In those last three months in Dubai an old colleague of Stan's contacted him to ask if he would represent a UK company selling software to teach English. The software was aimed at education and commerce. They talked it through, and Stan explained that he didn't feel he would be well received. Let me try to explain. Stan was born in India but grew up in the UK from the age of nine. He looked Indian, he was a British Citizen, he spoke like an Englishman, and he absolutely looked like an English gentleman in his Austin Reed suits, pristine white shirts, and silk ties. However, a huge part of the manual working population in Dubai are Indian, and in a lot of cases they are not well viewed or treated. I realise this is a sensitive subject, and I am trying my best to explain without offence.

Stan and John discussed different options and concluded that someone white British would be better suited to the role. After much discussion about the ideal candidate, they decided the person should be white, with English as their first language, and probably female. It was suggested that I might fit the bill!

We agreed that I would take on the role, but that we would return to the UK as a family and settle back there, and I would travel back to Dubai every six weeks for meetings and presentations. Stan had spent a lot of time away from his daughters, so this seemed like a good way of him spending more time with them, with the help of other members of the family.

The packing up commenced, and it was decided that instead of going straight back to the UK, we would use the Business Class ticket value to fly economy and do an around-the-world trip!

Our belongings left Dubai en route to the UK, and we moved out of our home to stay in a hotel in Dubai for three days before setting off on our adventure. Georgina had suffered with a lot of respiratory problems in the last six months of living in Dubai, but within 12 hours of leaving our house, the coughing stopped! When we looked back, we realised the house had been fumigated after the air conditioning broke, and we had been forced to move out briefly because it was overrun with cockroaches. The two incidents were probably linked, but we were all just grateful that Georgina was feeling better!

So, with a small case each, we set off, with Singapore, Bali, Darwin, Cairns, Sydney, Auckland, and Los Angeles just some of the stops. We did 13 flights in 33 days!!!

We did sightseeing tours, we had cocktails in Raffles, we stayed where Princess Diana had stayed in Bali, we saw incredible scenery and wildlife in Australia, we visited the Barrier Reef. One of the flights was over Ayers Rock/Uluru, and my tendency towards travel sickness didn't make it the best trip – particularly as we were in a very small plane! Thankfully, there was a lovely lady, probably in her sixties, sitting next to me, and I had Georgina on my lap. The next thing I knew, Georgina was off my lap and in this lady's arms having an amazing time, whilst I was throwing up! Not one of my finest moments, but everyone else enjoyed the flight.

We stayed in amazing hotels, one of which was the Kakadu Crocodile Hotel in the Kakadu National Park, and the hotel is the shape of a huge crocodile. We also spent time with dear family friends in Rotorua in New Zealand.

One of my favourite photographs from the trip was of all of us in bright red life jackets – you can just see Georgina's head sticking out of hers – when we went white water rafting.

The longest flight we took was from Auckland to Los Angeles, and there hadn't been a single hitch with accommodation until we got to L.A. Unfortunately, there are two hotels with incredibly similar names there: one is stunning, and the staff are great (we had stayed there before, so we knew); the lesser version had no air conditioning, no food, and very few staff. It didn't dampen the trip, though, as we had seen so many beautiful places, made amazing memories, and enjoyed the most incredible time. I think Sarah can remember these travels, but I'm not sure Georgina can.

Chapter: Four

We eventually arrived back in the UK, tired and tanned, having had the most amazing trip. After a couple of days to readjust, we started to look for our new home. In the 1990s, you could arrange mortgages differently from the way it is done today. In the weeks and months before leaving Dubai, we had sold our home in the UK and arranged mortgage finance, solicitors, etc, for a new home. We just didn't know where it was going to be!

We had asked various family members to carry out initial viewings for us, but so far nothing stood out. Estate agents sent detailed particulars of properties, and we had these sent to Stan's parents. One evening, we went through a pile of probably 50 properties! One in particular stood out to Stan.

We had been travelling for 33 days, so didn't have suits or business clothes with us. Everything was en route in the shipping container on its way to the UK. So, when we arranged a viewing of a beautiful old property which was in need of renovation, we were dressed in our jeans, shirts, and walking boots. The seller didn't think we were suitable buyers of his property, and he was stunned when we made an offer and explained that we would like to complete within 28 days as there was a container due to arrive with all our belongings in it.

Over the following four weeks, somehow we made it happen! Even on the day of completion, the seller still wasn't convinced that we could afford to buy their home. They had started to pack, but were still wary that everything would go ahead in just four weeks. So we ended up helping them move their belongings!

Stan could visualise how this old house could look like our new home, although I couldn't in the early stages. But over the next six months, the entire house was replastered, rewired, replumbed, and overhauled. And we lived in it whilst most of this work was going on. We used to joke that the front door was only shut at night when we went to bed and the continuous stream of tradesmen had left for the day. It was a massive project!

Stan was made redundant after 25 years with the same company, which was a real body blow for him, but he directed his energy and planning expertise into our home.

He was in charge of the house renovation; we both took care of the girls; and I started my new job travelling back to Dubai every six weeks to sell software. Travelling in the late 1990s was a lot easier than it is now. With the help of a friendly travel agent, flights and hotels would be booked, and I would plan a full week of appointments.

I met some fascinating people on these trips, and I could travel freely in Dubai, Abu Dhabi, and other parts of the Emirates, where I would demonstrate the software, which was partly in Arabic and partly in English. I visited banks, universities, and some major Dubai multinational companies, and no visit back there was ever the same. One visit coincided with my friend Catharine's 40th birthday, and it was a great chance to see friends from when we had lived there, but also for an amazing knees-up. I have to admit that I got on the plane home still drunk from the celebrations, as Catharine and her family know how to celebrate.

Back in England, our beautiful home was almost finished, but very sadly we didn't live there for long. In fact, it was sold within three years from when we moved in.

You might wonder why this was…

It all started one Sunday night. I was packing my bags to go to work down south on the Monday. After a year of travelling back and forth to Dubai, we realised that the venture hadn't turned out as we had all hoped, so Stan had helped me set up my own business in the UK as a freelance trainer. That night, I was making sure everything was sorted for the girls for school the next morning, while Stan was lying on the sofa, having felt quite out of sorts all day. He had been to the doctors the week before, as he seemed to be getting a lot of headaches. The doctor had given him painkillers and thought it was cluster headaches.

On that Sunday evening, Stan became very, very distressed and said he felt like someone was kicking his head like a football. He tried to walk but could hardly stand. I couldn't leave him like that, so I contacted the out-of-hours doctor and was told to take him to the local hospital. I managed to get him to the car, but I wasn't sure how I was going to get him into the building.

When we arrived, I managed to get Stan into a wheelchair and pushed him into the hospital. Everything changed from that point on.

We were seen by a doctor who wanted to give him even stronger painkillers. Stan was a larger-than-life character whose energy would fill the room when he walked in, but that evening he was slumped in a wheelchair, holding his head in his hands. I knew I couldn't take him home, so I tried to explain how Stan was normally! Eventually, the doctor agreed to send Stan for further investigations at another hospital half an hour away.

They gave him more painkillers and arranged for him to travel by ambulance. I went with him, as my daughters were with their grandmother, who was living with us at the time.

They did lots of tests and gave him drugs to help him sleep, but I stayed with him throughout, and his brother Tony came to be with us.

Just 48 hours later, we were sitting on a ward in one of the largest hospitals in the UK. It was only then that we were given the devasting diagnosis of a Grade 4 brain tumour. The consultant went on to say that surgery would be necessary the following day, otherwise Stan's life expectancy was probably only six weeks. Now, even 20 years on, I can't actually find the words to explain the devastating effect of that news. The consultant then explained what they planned to do, and Stan signed the consent forms.

The following day, Stan went into surgery and almost all of the tumour was removed. I went in to see him in the recovery room and was met by the most amazing nurse who was taking care of him. She explained that he had come through the surgery and that we now needed to make him comfortable and remove some of the wires and tubes that were attached to him. She asked if I wanted to watch or if I wanted to help. I wanted to help in any way I could just to get the Stan we all so loved back to being his usual self. But I can say, with tears pouring down my face, that we never really got him back to who he had been.

He underwent this massive surgery, chemotherapy and all the challenges that go with that, then radiotherapy with a Perspex mask, all to try and remove or shrink the tumour. And an amazing team of surgeons, consultants, nurses, friends, and family supported us through this really difficult time.

We also made memories when we could, when Stan was well enough. He still wanted to travel and go on holiday, so we made a trip to Gran Canaria, which I will never forget.

My mum and stepdad came from their home in Spain to Gran Canaria to spend time with us. But the experience of going through an airport with Stan in a wheelchair, at that point very poorly, was hard going. I was trying to help him, keep an eye on the girls, and not stress! Almost impossible.

However, we made it to Gran Canaria and to this massive hotel, but the size of the place just added to the challenges. Stan decided to go walkabout on his own one day. He just got up from the table and walked off. The only problem was he didn't have the faintest idea where he was!

Hours later, we were still frantically trying to find him in this massive complex. When we eventually found him, we all sat in the foyer, but he was so exhausted by the experience that he just couldn't walk any further. The hotel didn't have a wheelchair, and the airline had only provided one for use at the airport. So, in the end, we had to improvise. In the back office behind reception, we found a typist chair with wheels on, and that was what we used to get him back to our room. That was one of many long and emotional days.

I remember a group of us going to a Japanese restaurant in Birmingham to celebrate Stan's 50th birthday. By that point, he was struggling with his sight and mobility, but we managed an insane number of stairs to the restaurant and had the most amazing evening.

Stan had always been a planner! So, when he was able to, he continued to plan, and over the next few months he directed others to carry out his wishes, which included us moving house to something more manageable, in a local village with shops that he thought he would be able to walk to.

There weren't many properties on the market, and we needed to find something quickly.

One Sunday afternoon, I went into the local village where we were looking and bumped into an old school friend, Viv. She commented on how tired I looked, and I just broke down and told her about Stan and the fact we needed to find somewhere to live. She lived in the village herself and mentioned a house she knew that had been on the market but had been taken off recently. She told me which agents were dealing with it and suggested I ring them first thing Monday morning. I did.

The house was owned by a couple, but one wanted to sell and the other didn't. I explained our situation and asked if we could view the property, but I was told by the agents that they didn't think we would get a viewing. They said the lady worked shifts, but after a bit of pushing they agreed to ring her. It turned out she was going to be there that morning, so we arranged a viewing for an hour later to give me chance to get Stan ready.

Stan was really struggling with stairs at that stage, but he made it into the house, looked round the ground floor and through the kitchen window to the garden. He got upstairs and had a quick look and then made an offer on the spot, explaining why he wanted us to move. This whole process was exhausting for him, but he wanted to do it for us.

Over the next few months, we sold our beautiful home that we had worked so hard for and bought our new more manageable home. For various reasons, I ended up driving the big yellow van which was used to move our belongings the three miles to our new house. I think we made about ten trips in all, and by 6.30pm that evening we collapsed on the sofa, grateful and relieved that we had managed it. That was in November 2001.

Immediately, Stan started planning his next project – the garden! He wanted to create a beautiful garden with huge ponds with koi carp, seating areas, aviaries, and a summerhouse as a man cave with a big fridge and huge television.

This meant major excavation works in our much smaller back garden. I think Stan had the dimensions of the old garden in his head when he was planning this, as we had to keep scaling things back, and I can remember trying to make a scale drawing for him to explain why we couldn't fit in everything he was visualising.

However, the beautiful garden, with all its painted trellis, fish, birds, and two huge ponds filled with water lilies, was stunning, and there was a summerhouse with a huge television and fridge! This was the last project he bought to fruition.

Throughout all of Stan's planning, normal life needed to be maintained – the day-to-day of family life, including school. Except, nothing was normal! Every few days, I would be speaking to nurses at the hospital to check symptoms and changes in Stan. I would be the dispenser of his many tablets and medication. The man we all loved so much was so changed by his surgery and treatment.

Stan died, aged 50, in May 2002.

We gathered in his beautiful garden after his funeral, where we celebrated his life, and one of his dear friends recited a poem about his precious garden as we remembered an incredible husband, father, son, brother, and friend. There are no words to describe the devastation felt by all his family and friends.

I became a widow at 34, and our daughters became my reason to go on.

Chapter: Five

I can clearly recall sitting in Stan's favourite chair, swaying back and forth, not knowing what to do, how I felt, or how I was supposed to live without him.

I knew I needed to stay strong for Sarah and Georgina, but also for Stan's mum. I will be brutally honest and admit that sometimes I got it right, and other times I didn't. I just had to start by doing the basics of getting out of bed in the morning and making sure the girls were up, dressed, fed, and taken to school. Sounds simple, but in the early days I couldn't manage anything else. I had promised Stan that I would take care of our girls and his mum, and I tried to do that through all the turmoil and upset.

I don't think there is a book that tells you how exactly to cope with grief, and this book isn't intended to either. What I share here is my own experience of grief and loss.

I did go for counselling at my doctor's surgery, for a block of hourly sessions for six weeks, and that gave me a safe space to share how I really felt, which was lost, angry, tired, confused, incredibly sad, and a whole lot of other emotions. I think my overwhelming feeling was why I had only got to spend such a small amount of time with the person I'd wanted to grow old with. I felt so uncertain about how I would cope bringing our daughters up without him by my side. I also questioned myself and whether I could have done more to help Stan. But medical staff, family, and friends, at different times reassured me that we had all done what we could.

My daughters were 17 and seven when they lost their dad. Sarah was at college, and Georgina was still at primary school. Both college and school provided much needed support and just kept an eye on all of us in a loving and kind way.

Inevitably, there are people who just don't know what to say or how to react to you in these situations, but I felt held and supported while I tried to be the best mum I could be. Like I said before, I didn't get it all right, but I know I tried my best. There were so many things to sort out, when just the simple things seemed more than enough to cope with.

We all grieve in different ways, and there were many times when I felt completely alone. A dear friend, Mary, suggested getting a dog, as she said that it might help with the grief and provide some much-needed distraction for my girls. My daughters thought this was a great idea. We'd had dogs before, but when Stan became ill, they'd been looked after and adopted by friends.

Mary had a friend who bred Jack Russells, and there was another litter due soon, so it was agreed that we would just go and take a look. There was a litter of six, all different colours – and of course, there was a runt.

I think it would be fair to say 'Alfie' picked us! He was the runt of the litter and made a beeline for Georgina.

The pups were too young to leave their mum, so the following Sunday we went back to see them again, and Alfie stepped forward yet again. I had been chatting privately to the breeder about the timescale to pick up Alfie. We arranged that when he was ready, I would just say we were visiting and then surprise the girls and say we could take him home! Alfie was black, white, and tan, and he looked like a Doberman pup.

After a few weeks, he came home with us, and the joys of having a puppy soon created a distraction from everything else. We had a lovely dining table and chairs, but the dining chair legs were never the same again after Alfie arrived! He was mischievous but full of love, and he was happy to share that love with our family of three.

After a while, we thought we should go to puppy training lessons (I would say human training sessions). So, once a week for six weeks, we drove about 20 miles for these sessions, and during these times we laughed, and we cried. The first evening, Alfie was the smallest there, and the largest were two huge standard poodles, who were definitely better behaved than him. Somehow, Alfie did get his certificate at the end of the six weeks, but he was always a bit of a free spirit! Nevertheless, he took happily to his role as protector – something he did for 16 years.

As I mentioned, at that time I had my own training business, but this was no longer viable because I didn't want to be away from the girls. So, I took on a part-time job in a shop in the village that sold cookery items and housewares. It was good just to be around different people and out of the house.

After a while, I wanted to do something that used my skills a bit more, so I moved on and got a part-time job working in a solicitor's office, which I found fascinating. In my early twenties I had worked for an estate agent and had always had an interest in buying and selling property. Actually, I don't think I want to add up the number of times I have moved house, bought, and sold property in the last 30 years.

That first year after Stan died, there were a number of family celebrations, including Georgina's first holy communion and Sarah's 18th birthday. We were glad to have events to celebrate, but it was incredibly tough without Stan there.

At times I felt incredibly supported by family and friends, but at other times I felt completely alone just trying to stay sane. Watching someone you love go through any illness is hard, but seeing Stan go through all his surgery and treatments had been horrendous. I couldn't believe how brutal everything had been.

I wanted to find something gentle and soothing to do that would make me feel better, so I enrolled on an aromatherapy course at a local holistic centre. This gave me a focus one day a week during term time.

I really enjoyed being with lovely people, and it was great to do something different and use my brain so it didn't go to mush, which was how it felt at times. I loved everything about it... until it came to doing case studies. I was fine with female clients, but not male ones. It just made me feel incredibly uneasy on so many different levels.

With hard work and perseverance, I finally passed my exams and gained my qualification.

A friend of mine suggested that going for a Reiki treatment might be good for me. I had been for massage for lower back problems, so I saw no reason not to try it.

I can clearly remember those first Reiki sessions. I usually fell asleep, wrapped under blankets, with beautiful music playing. I felt safe. I didn't need to take any clothes off, I just snuggled down, and I always came away feeling a heck of a lot better than when I had gone in.

As I slowly began to rebuild my life, friends would tell me it was time to stop wearing black, which I had done out of respect for Stan. I know this sounds old-fashioned, but I think for me it was part of the process.

I had felt really supported by the church which Stan, his parents, and family had attended for many, many years. So I became a eucharist minister, taking communion to the sick in their homes or nursing homes, and this took up most of my Sunday afternoons. Georgina used to come with me and try to brighten the day for those we were visiting.

One Sunday afternoon, though, we were involved in a road traffic accident on our way home. That really shook me and put an end to the Sunday afternoon visiting.

After a couple of years on my own, I was being gently nudged by family and friends to get out and meet people. In some cases, a few friends were more direct in encouraging me to 'meet someone'. The same friend Mary, who had suggested we get a dog, also suggested a blind date. She'd had a really tough time and her marriage had ended, but she had found love again and thought I could do the same.

At a golf dinner, Mary was seated next to her new husband, and on the other side of her was Mike, who was to become my blind date a couple of weeks later! I was pretty adamant that I wasn't ready for this, but my friend had other ideas. Bless her.

I explained to the girls that I was just going out for a drink with Mary, her husband Tom, and Mike. But I was a nervous wreck. I got dressed and left the house, only then realising that I was about half an hour early. However, I knew if I went back into the house, I would not go out again!

To kill some time, I decided to stop off at a local pub on my way and bumped into someone I used to work with. He commented that I looked very smart but very nervous! When I explained that I was insanely anxious at the thought of dating, he bought me a very large gin and tonic and told me I would be fine.

When I got to my friend's house, Mike was rolling around on the grass in the back garden with their dog. He got up and brushed himself off, and we got on like a house on fire from then on.

It didn't all go swimmingly, though; the backlash from family on all fronts wasn't much fun. Some felt it was too soon; others didn't like the fact I was widowed. I could go on, but I won't. Mike didn't know much about me and my life at this point, other than that I had been widowed and had two daughters.

We realised very quickly that we shared friends and acquaintances, and on that first date in a local pub, we were both greeted by one, Bruce, who knew us both but for very different reasons. Bruce had been a friend of my dad for years. It was very strange.

That time was great in so many ways, but also very challenging in others. I felt loved, but I also didn't want to upset my daughters by making a life with someone new. Somehow, we weathered those storms of the early days in our relationship, and I continued to rebuild my life and support my daughters. It wasn't easy, and I know I made mistakes.

During this quite stressful time, I decided to go for more Reiki and massage sessions, and I enjoyed it so much that I felt I would like to learn Reiki. Little did I realise at that point the help that it would provide in the coming years.

There are many different types of Reiki, but I learned the more traditional Usui Reiki, which is a Japanese form of energy healing for stress reduction and relaxation that also promotes healing. Reiki treats the whole person. Learning Reiki was something for me, and to help me feel better.

In 2008, not long after celebrating my 40th birthday, my dear stepdad John was diagnosed with pancreatic cancer. My mum and John had retired to Spain, and Mum needed help taking care of him.

My daughters and Mike were supportive of me going out to Spain, so I made a few trips in the short months before he died. I just felt I needed to support my mum and John's daughter Caroline, who came out to see him a few days before he died. Those phone calls to Caroline to explain how poorly her dad was were hard, but necessary. And before he passed away, John got to see Caroline and his newest grandson, who was only six weeks old.

I have written recently about bereavement in a collaboration book called *Beautifully Broken*. I am not frightened of death; I think that comes from having lost so many close family and friends. But I made a promise to John that I would take care of Mum, and I have done so. They had a deep love for one another and were a very special couple. They had first married back in 1961 but divorced a couple of years later. My mum met and married my dad, had me and my sister, then that marriage eventually fell apart. In the meantime, John had married again and had Caroline. In the early 1990s, Mum and John remarried – their love for each other was so strong and had withstood the test of time.

In 2012, my mum had her own health scare when she was back visiting us in the UK. Although Mum had settled in Spain, she still visited at least a couple of times a year. She was offered a routine mammogram which sadly highlighted a tumour, and she was stunned to receive a diagnosis of breast cancer. Her own mother had been diagnosed with cancer in her early seventies.

My dear mum had a mastectomy, and thankfully didn't require any radiotherapy or chemotherapy. I tried my best to support her both physically and emotionally but should probably admit that she definitely wasn't an easy patient!

Chapter: Six

At that point in April 2012, my own life was pretty stressful.

It all began when I took unwell and was diagnosed with shingles, due to a very unpleasant rash around my neck and throat. I was given anti-viral medication by an out-of-hours GP, but a couple of weeks after this, I developed a sore lump under my tongue. The shingles disappeared but the lump didn't. I booked an appointment with my own GP, who told me not to worry and that the lump would go away in a few weeks. But the pain in my mouth grew increasingly worse.

I had a routine dental hygienist appointment a week later, at which I mentioned the horrendous discomfort I was experiencing. I was due to go on holiday in a few days, so they managed to get me seen that day by the dentist who was on duty. I was told to take antibiotics, rinse with mouthwash, and to enjoy my holiday. The dentist I saw said to make an appointment for after my holiday.

I booked an appointment for two weeks later with my own dentist, who I had been seeing for over 20 years. I then took their advice and trusted that my sore and swollen tongue would soon be back to normal, and I had a great holiday.

On my return, my own dentist examined me and immediately knew something wasn't right. I was referred to our local hospital, where I was booked in for what I assumed to be an initial consultation. Due to the increased pain and swelling, and the reduced movement of my tongue, the registrar was unable to carry out the initial examination herself. Instead, she asked if I could wash my hands and attempt to lift up my tongue to show her the affected area.

I will never forget the alarmed look on her face before she asked for me to be seen by another consultant downstairs. I was already feeling tired and weary after what had been a very long day of waiting, but I made my way downstairs, innocently unaware that the worst was yet to come.

The pain that seared through my body as the nurse took the biopsies was almost unbearable! The memory still sends shudders through me now. I remember thinking that I would rather cut my own tongue off than repeat that vile procedure. I wiped the tears from my eyes, took a deep breath, and composed myself before she repeated the procedure for the second, and then the third time!

A week later, rested and (just about!) recovered from the ordeal of the biopsies, I went back to the hospital for my results. I can't remember the exact words, but basically, I was told I had a squamous cell carcinoma of the tongue – cancer of the tongue. I'll be honest, it didn't really come as a huge surprise to me. It did, however, come as a massive shock to my partner Mike, who had come with me to the appointment for moral support. I saw the colour drain from his face, and he looked like he had been hit by a tank!

I was 44 years old, a mum to two gorgeous girls – by then aged 27 and 17 – a partner, a daughter, a sister, and a friend. In what felt like a blink of an eye, I was now also a cancer patient. Cancer of the tongue is normally associated with heavy drinkers and smokers, and in some cases HPV (Human Papillomavirus). In my case, I felt wholeheartedly that it had been brought on by stress.

After that, everything happened so quickly.

One minute I was being told of my diagnosis, the next I was being told about the huge and very risky operation that was to follow. I tried my hardest to absorb the fact that they planned to do a neck dissection – a cut from under my left ear, all the way under my chin, and halfway up to my right ear – taking lymph nodes to check if the cancer had spread beyond my tongue. Then they would sever my tongue, taking enough away to completely remove the tumour. After that, they would perform a skin graft from my left arm, which would include a nerve. This would be used to reconnect my tongue and the nerve down my left arm, which would enable me to still use my left arm and, 'all being well', enable me to be able to learn to swallow, eat, and speak again!

The final part of the surgery jigsaw was where they would take flesh from my stomach to refill the area in my arm that had been removed. I joke about this part now, as I always refer to it as my added bonus of a tummy tuck!

Now, it all sounds simple when it's written down like that, but the enormity of the surgery would only be realised a couple of months later.

From the ward where I was diagnosed, I walked in disbelief to the breast cancer ward – yes, my mum and I were seen in the same hospital – where I explained that I might need a bit more help supporting Mum, as I had just received devastating news of my own. The staff were amazingly supportive.

I remember going home that afternoon in a state of shock. I was scared for myself and what was ahead of me, but more for my family and how this would impact upon them.

When I was first diagnosed, I was heavier than I would have liked. I tried to stay positive, but sadly there are many risks with this type of surgery, and I'd been told I would have to learn to eat and swallow again and speak! You initially lose weight with the worry and stress of the diagnosis, and then you physically struggle to eat for sometimes weeks or months after the surgery. I was not able to have a Percutaneous Endoscopic Gastrostomy (PEG) feeding tube because of my earlier colon surgery.

At this point, I want to acknowledge the most amazing team who took care of me at Russells Hall and New Cross Hospitals. That includes surgeons, anaesthetists, an oncologist, a speech therapist, physiotherapist, radiographer, nutritionist, and the most amazing clinical nurse specialists and staff on the wards.

It may sound like a strange thing to say, but I had to trust with all my heart that they would help me get through this whole experience, and I kept that thought every single day. I knew that I would be in the very safe hands of the experts, but unfortunately there was one part they couldn't help me with – the part I dreaded the most. Telling my beautiful daughters. Georgina was taking her A-levels at the time that all of this was happening.

I can vividly remember a meeting with my consultant at which he reiterated very strongly the need to tell family and close friends about my diagnosis. I agreed I would… as soon as I had a plan.

Following on from the diagnosis, I had CT and MRI scans so that the surgeons could pinpoint the area of the tumour. The MRI experience was one I will never forget. I was looked after by a lovely gentleman who suggested I should imagine I was somewhere beautiful, not in a noisy MRI scanner. I imagined that I was lying on a sun lounger on my favourite beach in the south of France, and I got through the MRI. If you can believe it, I actually fell asleep!

The planning continued at the hospital, and I did eventually let the information out, but not until my youngest daughter had finished her last exam.

One valuable piece of advice I had been given by my lead surgeon was to keep those who loved and would support me incredibly close, and not allow those who I felt would not support my decisions near me whilst I was going through the surgery and treatment. This may sound harsh, but it makes perfect sense – you need as much love and support as you can muster, and as few worriers and stress providers.

The time between diagnosis and surgery was spent trying to function as if everything was fine, trying to live a normal day-to-day life, but I was in a lot of pain. I concentrated on writing my will and setting up a power of attorney for financial matters as well as for health and wellbeing. The health/wellbeing power of attorney is your opportunity to plan who can act on your behalf if you are no longer able to communicate or make decisions for yourself. I took specialist legal advice on this.

Finally, the time came for my surgery, along with potentially 17 days of recovery in hospital, with the possibility that I might not be able to speak again and might lose the use of my left arm!

I was admitted to hospital early in the morning the day before my surgery and, miraculously, I managed to sleep that night. The ward I spent that first night on specialised in head and neck surgery, and the staff were incredibly kind and supportive even before the operation had taken place.

On the day of my surgery, I wrote in a beautiful notebook gifted by my friend Judy:

12th June, 2012

6.25am – washed, gowned, and ready.

I have every faith in the team looking after me. They have explained what they plan to do, and I am positive that all will be well.

My thoughts, as ever, are with all my family and friends, but I know their thoughts are with me.

I am strong.

That first notebook would be one of three that would become my lifeline in hospital, helping me to get my point across to everyone around me when I was unable to speak.

When I woke up in the recovery ward after 11 hours of very complicated surgery, I was incredibly frightened, and I couldn't speak! I had a tracheotomy – an opening created at the front of my neck so a tube could be inserted into the windpipe (trachea) to help me breathe – and I looked like I had hit a brick wall. I was surrounded by nurses who were checking wires and tubes and taking vital observations. It was incredibly scary, and I wanted to communicate with more than just my eyes! But my face was completely disfigured by the surgery, so facial expressions were completely useless at that point.

Eventually, I got them to understand that I wanted a piece of paper and a pen so that I could communicate. They found a clipboard, paper, and pen, and I could then begin to express what I wanted. I was as high as a kite on morphine and other drugs at that stage. As you know, it wasn't the first time I had been in a recovery room, and I remembered the most amazing nurse who had helped my husband. That recollection and insight meant I understood so much more of what was happening to me there.

I couldn't use my left arm at all, as it was so heavily bandaged from that part of the surgery. But I felt relieved that I had survived the operation, and I was eventually transferred onto a ward.

My first night on the ward was horrendous. There was an elderly lady in the bed across the ward, who thought I was her daughter. She kept calling out to me and asking the nurses why I wasn't speaking to her. This went on for hours, but I couldn't speak to anyone, no matter how much I wanted to!

The following day, things weren't going according to plan. My new tongue was dying, and it was then that it came to light that the first operation hadn't worked and the nerve into my arm had not been connected.

So, off I went, back into surgery for a further 11 hours!

Everything initially progressed well, and this time the tongue was healing, until a few days later they realised that I had a blockage in my neck. This resulted in my third major operation three days later.

18th June, 2012

ENOUGH!!! I am in charge of what you do to me, I want to know what's happening! I wanted to scream, but I couldn't make a sound.

My frustration reached boiling point as I ripped the feeding tube out of my nose. I couldn't take it any more. I couldn't speak or swallow, let alone scream out loud. But I also couldn't stop the rage that had been building inside me for far too long.

I had endured 22 hours of surgery over two days, only to find out a few days later that I had a blockage in my neck which required yet another operation. The third visit to surgery was a turning point in my life! I felt with every bone in my body that I was incredibly lucky to have survived that trip to theatre, but made a conscious decision that when I did finally come around from the anaesthetic, enough was enough.

My entire life had consisted of me not speaking up, being scared of voicing my opinions, feeling like my voice didn't matter, or being very quickly silenced if what I was saying didn't want to be heard.

Now, here I was, literally with no voice! It was in that very moment that I knew something had to change. I remember the look of horror on the nurses' faces as they tried to calm me down and reinsert the tube. They must have thought I had lost the plot. Despite being drugged up on copious amounts of pain relief and knowing that I had a long road of recovery, I also knew there were going to be big changes in my life. It was time for me to finally find my voice and speak up for myself. My only means of communication at that point was to write down what I needed or wanted to say.

It seemed crazy that only 12 weeks prior to the operation, I had been living a relatively 'normal' life. I'd had my fair share of good and bad times, but my old life and face were no longer recognisable! I had no idea if either would ever be the same again, and that was extremely scary.

I understand that this was also an incredibly hard time for my family. My mum, cousin, partner, and daughters, all visited me in the first few days, and the sight must have been shocking. I can only imagine how awful those visits were for them. But I wanted to prove to each and every person that saw me that I was strong enough to get through this and that I would make a full recovery.

The days were filled with all the usual checks, drugs, and inspections of my wounds, and the nights were horrendous! I had one night when I listened continually to the album *Anthems*, by Russell Watson, which was one of the soundtracks that was used for the Olympic Games in 2012. I was so frightened that if I shut my eyes, I wouldn't wake up again.

Russell Watson had survived a brain tumour and returned to his singing career, so my thoughts were that if he could do it, so could I!

A couple of years after my surgery, Mike took me to Preston. I know, very glamorous! But we went to see Russell Watson in concert at the Preston Guild Hall. It was amazing to hear him sing live. When there was an interval, Russell mingled with the audience. He didn't know how important his music had been to me, but I desperately wanted to shake his hand. We were sitting in the middle of a row of people, but I was determined to get to him even if I had to clamber over the entire row. I did shake his hand, and when I hear tracks from that album, I'm grateful he survived his cancer and that his music helped me survive mine.

I also felt the power of music with another track – *Angels*, by Robbie Williams. (As I am writing this, I am listening to that song again.) I was surrounded by angels whilst I was in hospital, because that is the view I had of the most amazing team who took care of me. The medics don't see themselves as angels, but I most certainly did. There were a few not so pleasant experiences, but I have learnt that holding onto those scary situations and the anger I felt only hurts me now.

It was probably three or four days after my surgery when I actually saw myself in the mirror. There are no words to describe how I felt and how different I looked. I could hardly lift my head up properly for many, many months – not out of shame; it just wasn't physically possible.

After 17 days in hospital – one of which nearly saw me sectioned – I was finally allowed to go home! I am thankful every day for the two friends – Sharon, a legal executive, and Jude, a counsellor – who rushed to the hospital to vouch for me after I managed to text them to say I desperately needed their help. I was having some bad reactions to the morphine, including hallucinations, and feeling that I wasn't in my body! One night, I felt I was floating round the ward, completely separate to my body, which I could see lying in the bed below me.

The nights were the hardest, loneliest times. The staff on the wards were amazing, but they were busy, and not being able to communicate was almost like being a prisoner.

I was writing all this down and trying to explain how trau-matised I felt by the surgery and many other events in my life. My mum, probably due to fear, thought I had lost the plot. But I hadn't! I was just trying to vocalise on paper the level of distress that I was feeling, and I also had things I wanted to say in case I didn't survive!

Sharon explained to the medics and to my mum that I de-finitely was of sane mind, as I had put all my affairs in order before my surgery, and Jude explained that I had been going to see her for counselling. The reaction to her comments was that they hadn't realised I had mental health issues. I didn't; I went for counselling!

In total, I wrote in three notebooks in the 17 days I was in hospital. The first one had whole pages of scribbles and paragraphs that didn't make sense. There were pages where I was pleading for pain relief and to be discharged. There were also pages of me explaining to my family what was happening when they weren't with me, and some of that was incredibly scary.

One day, when my youngest daughter came to see me, we had a whole conversation in my journal, and she wrote how proud she was of me. I also wrote about my life and the many experiences of taking care of people, and now finding myself needing to be cared for.

Sometimes we don't acknowledge to ourselves, let alone anyone else, how we are truly feeling. In the time before I got my ability to speak back, those notebooks were literally my lifeline.

Each day followed the regular routine of observations, checking my wounds, copious amounts of painkillers, steroids, and antibiotics, and sleeping. Then, when I was awake, watching the clock waiting for visitors to arrive.

I was on anti-coagulant injections to avoid blood clots, as I couldn't move much from my bed. I decided I could maybe help avoid clots if I kept moving my body, so I lay in bed stretching and moving what bits I could, including circling my ankles and bending my knees. That was probably another time when they thought they had a nutter on the ward!

I had physiotherapy to get movement back in my arms, but also to actually get me moving at all after the trauma of the surgery.

After a couple of days, I was also visited by one of the speech and language therapists. She explained that I needed to be determined and to practise if I was going to regain my speech. She explained that trying to form the letters of the alphabet and counting numbers would be a good place to start. So, I did! My whole face was misshapen, but I knew I had to try.

Day after day, I sat there forming the words. I don't know how many days it took before I actually made a recognisable sound, as the hours went by in a blur, with me still writing down what I needed and how I felt.

I also had to learn to swallow, so I was given water which had a thickening agent added to it. It was a case of just trying and seeing if I could manage it, and eventually I didn't feel like I was drowning.

Eating, though, was a whole different experience. Whilst in hospital, I was initially fed through a tube in the very early days post-surgery. Then I was given ready-to-drink, high calorie nutritional supplement shakes. They don't taste great, but that doesn't really come into it at that stage. After a few days, I then had pureed food, and very slowly food with more texture.

When I was finally discharged after 17 days, I think it was a huge relief for everyone! During my time in hospital, family and friends had supported my girls and Mike in so many different ways, and he sent out regular emails to them to update them on my progress.

On that first day home, I wanted to sit and eat with my family. And I wanted a curry! Yes, that's right; I wanted something with flavour. Everyone enjoyed their food with texture and flavour; mine, however, had been pureed in a blender!

Learning to eat and swallow food was a slow process, involving trial and error, and each day was different – both in hospital and once I made it home. Some days I could swallow food with more texture than on other days. I found *Brenda's Easy to Swallow Cookbook*, by Brenda Brady, a great help, and the recipes included some from very well-known chefs. This was published in January 2009.

I kept spreadsheets to keep track of my medications, but this sheet was also used to mark down what I had managed to eat. That could simply have been a ridiculously small amount of scrambled egg, or a little bowl of homemade soup.

I was on lots of medication, which had different effects on me and how I felt. But I reckoned that at least if it was all written down, if I couldn't remember if I had taken the medication, my family could check and keep an eye on things.

This may sound strange, but I had to *want* to eat as well as being physically able to do it. My family were incredibly supportive, and they would look for different foods that I could try. I started off with very simple things, but soon realised that some foods I just couldn't do. Even 10 years on, there are certain foods that are a no-go, and a big part of my journey has been about acceptance. My tastebuds did recover, but for quite a few months nothing tasted quite right, and certain food or drinks just didn't pass my lips.

I mentioned the problem with swallowing, because having had the oral surgery and tracheotomy, the throat area was incredibly sore and inflamed. As a result, I am still a fan of mugs of honey and lemon to soothe my throat, and I know if I have spent all day chatting or on the phone, my throat is sore. On a rare occasion now, my speech can be slurred when I am really tired.

I recovered quite well from the surgery, and my wounds started to heal, but after a short period of time – only a matter of weeks – I started my radiotherapy treatment. In my case, this was to be undertaken every day for six weeks, with the weekends off for good behaviour – only joking. You need the weekends to catch your breath and sleep.

The team at the Deanesly Centre were amazing. The scariest part was having to wear a mask made of a mesh which is moulded to the shape of your face. At different times, I did look up information on the internet – some of it was helpful, but other things just filled me with dread. I didn't look up any information about the mask-making process, but I had a friend who did.

The mask is made to hold your head and neck still and in exactly the right position. This helps make your treatment as accurate and effective as possible. The mask fits tightly, but should not be uncomfortable, and you can breathe normally while you are wearing it.

It starts out a mesh-like fabric which is wet and then shaped over your face – not a pleasant experience, if I'm really honest. This is used each day to make sure that the radiotherapy is hitting the correct spots – in my case, both sides of my neck and my tongue. The mask is also used to attach you to the radiotherapy bed!

My first experience of this was horrendous, but I became more accepting of it and began counting down the days to the end of my six-week treatment. A few years after my treatment had finished, I found my green mesh mask in the spare room. I took great pleasure in stamping on it and throwing it away, finally ready to let it go!

The radiotherapy is cumulative, and it keeps on working in your body well after the six weeks; in fact, it can stay in your body for many years. Every day after my treatment, I would rest, and sometimes sleep. And our trusty little Jack Russell, Alfie, would lie on my feet and guard me as I rested.

My cousin had planned her wedding on 21st September, 2012, and I was adamant I wanted to attend. But as my last two radiotherapy treatments were both on the 31st of August, the hospital staff really doubted that I would be well enough to go to the wedding. I, however, had no doubts! I was going, even if that meant buying a big, beautiful hat to cover up my scars.

In the end, we did go to the wedding, and it was a beautiful day. I wore scarves to hide my scars and burns, but I wouldn't have missed it for the world.

Chapter: Seven

After my surgery, and during my treatment, I asked my partner Mike if he would take me to London. And we actually did this twice! We went to see *Mamma Mia* on one trip, and the closing ceremony of the Paralympics at Wembley for the second one! Coldplay were part of the closing ceremony, and I even found my squeaky voice to join in. It was incredible!

I was really struggling with exhaustion at the time when we did the Paralympics, so Mike decided a wheelchair would be the best option. And he walked miles and miles, pushing me along without complaint. I think I would have felt really out of place at any other event, but not on that occasion.

The burns around my neck, from the radiotherapy, were very visible and painful so scarves became a vital part of my wardrobe. At this point I had special impregnated dresses that you cut like a sewing pattern, so that you could get them to fit around the neck area, which was red raw from the radiotherapy. I have always worn scarves, but now they were a necessity rather than a pretty addition.

I have some great pictures of me in red, white, and blue, taken outside Wembley, and some incredible pictures of the inside of the stadium that night. Many years later, I went there again to see Adele in concert. There is something amazing about the energy in a huge arena, with so many people there to enjoy every moment.

After the closing ceremony and an incredible day, Mike had to push me all the way back to the hotel! But the adventure and all that excitement kept me going for weeks afterwards. Part of my enjoyment was seeing sportsmen and women with disabilities who could do amazing things and be amazing people. It was inspiring.

I think the fact that I so wanted things to look forward to was hugely important and played a big part in my recovery.

After being discharged from hospital, I was seen in the outpatient's department to see how I was getting on, to review medication, and to check for any problems with the various wounds. These visits started off weekly, and slowly got to monthly, and then six monthly, but I always felt supported – even when things weren't going quite to plan. You build up a rapport with the consultants and nursing staff, and I found that incredibly reassuring.

For a while, I also attended a support group specifically for head and neck patients. It was only for two hours once a month, but it provided reassurance and gave me an opportunity to see the amazing clinical nurse specialists and other patients going through similar experiences. Some had just gone through surgery and treatment, while others had survived many, many years and wanted to share the fact that they were still there and getting on with life.

We also compared notes on what we were managing to eat or drink. Even now, ten years on, there are certain foods that are just not a good idea, either because of the risk of choking or the clag factor! (How sticky or gloopy certain foods are.) I was also supported by a local lymphoedema clinic, who taught me how to massage my neck in order to lessen the fluid retention there.

It became important to me to keep trying different foods, and I had some good days and some horrendous days! But I just kept trying. After the surgery was actually easier than after the radiotherapy, because the burns are not only on the outside of your body but also on the inside.

Mike and I also had sessions with a counsellor who was used to dealing with head and neck patients and the specific problems that can arise from this kind of surgery.

I mentioned earlier that by then I had trained in both Aromatherapy and Reiki. These two holistic healing modalities played a huge role in my recovery, together with an unshakeable determination to get through whatever surgery and treatments were needed. I also wanted to lessen the number of drugs I was taking.

I went from taking oral morphine, as well as other painkillers, to morphine patches. Then, over a period of four months, I managed to wean myself off the morphine altogether. There are times when you need the painkillers in order to be able to function, and this can be hard for people to understand.

My Reiki teacher, Susie Gessey, also supported me in so many different ways, including sending healing to me whilst I was in hospital and then visiting me at home when I was discharged. Another way was an affirmation that we agreed upon: I am healed, and I am free to be me. I said these few powerful words over and over in my head hundreds of times whilst lying in hospital, as well as moving my face and mouth to form letters and words.

While I was in hospital, incredibly scared and in a lot of pain, one night I realised that I had a book about Reiki on my phone, and I managed to read it and to do some of the healing exercises.

Reiki is not the easiest holistic therapy to explain, but in very simple terms it aids the body's own ability to heal and can help to relax the body.

I imagined that I was sending healing to my arm, as I had had a bad reaction to some of the dressings. The wound was open so I could look at it, and it wasn't pretty, believe me. However, I knew that without this radical surgery, I didn't have a chance. Dressings which I didn't have a bad reaction to were impregnated with silver and honey, which are used in plastic surgery, and they were amazing for my arm.

I also knew from past experiences of seeing loved ones in hospital that staying positive would definitely help me get through.

However, a cancer diagnosis doesn't just affect the person with the disease. It affects all those around them – I know this from my own experiences – and there is a sense of helplessness.

I can remember one day after radiotherapy, my skin was so tight at my neck that I thought it would burst, and I knew that did happen to some people. The pain was indescribable, and I just wanted to scream. I did, and that screaming was directed at someone I loved dearly. It wasn't their fault; they didn't understand how I felt. They wanted to understand but couldn't. I tried to keep my outbursts to a minimum, but sometimes in those situations you just can't help it.

I had a slightly more amusing return journey from radiotherapy with my friend Sharon, when I was swearing like a trooper. I am not really someone who swears, but oh my goodness, that day I turned the air blue. My friend was open-mouthed with shock! But I just needed to voice how awful I felt and to let out some of my anger at the pain and discomfort.

I am a good project manager, and overnight I became the most important project I had ever taken on! I used to have a notebook with me at every single hospital appointment, which meant I didn't forget anything, and I could go back and refer to my notes later if I hadn't taken some information in.

During my recovery period, I was contacted by a friend I had previously worked with. She had changed jobs and was now selling natural products as part of a network marketing company. The company had medically qualified advisers who would provide guidance for particular customers, if required.

My friend sent them the graphic photos of my scars and wounds, and an explanation of what I was going through. This help and support also proved invaluable, and I still use some of those products now, even ten years on. Some things worked and others didn't, but I overwhelmingly wanted to feel better and get on with my life, so I was willing to give anything a try.

I am grateful every day for having that mindset and determination. Don't get me wrong, I'm not always happy and smiley, because life brings other challenges. But I have a tendency to dust myself off and step forwards again, even though that is harder on some days than others.

Being able to travel and spend time by the sea or ocean has provided opportunities for my body to heal. My daughters laugh at me and say, 'Mum thinks everything can be healed by sea air.' It probably doesn't, but spending time out in nature is something that certainly helps me.

It also encouraged me to look forward. In my experience, having something to look forward to – a visit to a special place or event – helps you focus and gives you something to aim for.

In the years that followed my diagnosis, treatment, and recovery, Mike and I were lucky enough to be able to travel. He resigned from his job to help take care of me, and I will always be incredibly grateful for his support. I am not sure he has ever really got over it.

We travelled to many different parts of France by car, as I found flying painful around my face, neck, and jaw, and for a long time I was very aware and embarrassed by my scars.

A few years ago, a friend looked at my family tree as a gift for my 50th birthday. I knew a little bit of family history but nothing of much substance. One of the many facts that came out was that I have ancestors who were stonemasons, so maybe that's where my fascination for buildings comes from. I love a medieval village or cathedral, and I've been lucky enough to visit stunning places in France, Italy, and

Spain. In times of distress, I have often found myself in church, lighting candles for those I love. It is only very recently that I found I could light a candle for myself!! I suggest you give it a try.

Our trips to France by car enabled us to bring lots of things back with us. In our case, not crates of wine, but ridiculous amounts of olive oil and lavender honey. We used to go to the same producers year after year. We also went to visit a beautiful essential oil distillery high up in the mountains near Grasse, which is famous for its perfumeries.

I have a love of nature, and something very beautiful that is created by Mother Earth is crystals. Since my illness, I have found a love and greater understanding of the very healing energy from crystals. I wear crystal jewellery, and every piece I have has a therapeutic property that has aided my healing. Sometimes you are drawn to specific colours, like soothing greens, or soft and gentle pinks, or reds for strength. You might not really know why you are drawn to wear a particular colour, but it just feels right.

After my radiotherapy treatment had finished, a lovely lady I had met, who did hair and makeup, suggested I have a makeover. At that point, my scars were still very visible, and I struggled to lift my head up. Looking at myself in the mirror wasn't something I enjoyed.

She also asked me about clothes, what I liked wearing, and what was my normal day-to-day clothing. I found this quite a difficult question to answer. My wardrobe had plenty of pinstriped suits and dark colours for legal meetings and funerals, along with jeans and long-sleeved tops (I was very conscious of the scar on my left arm and the line where they took the nerve, which is about six inches long and a centimetre across). I also wore lots of scarves to hide the scars of the neck dissection. There was a little colour in my wardrobe, but not much. She helped me to see that I could cover some of my very visible scars, and also showed me clothing shapes that would be flattering. The make-up part was really strange as I didn't want to look at myself because I felt like a bit of freak. But she helped me to find colours that made me look better, rather than draining out the bit of colour I had.

At that point, I had also lost a lot of weight; at my lowest point, I was just under eight stone. I'm 10 stone 6lb now, and quite happy with that. Losing weight when you are poorly isn't difficult, but putting it back on again took determination.

Over the following few years, there were some amazing trips and family celebrations both in the UK, France, and Spain, but also some tough times, too. My experience of the last ten years has been learning to appreciate and hold onto the good times and the memories you create in order to get through the tough stuff.

Chapter: Eight

In 2016, my eldest daughter Sarah married the love of her life, Shammie, and our beautiful granddaughter Sophie arrived. Sometimes the arrival of a new member of the family can be around the same time as the departure of another. And 2016 was also the year I lost my dad.

He had survived many health challenges, including heart surgery, and his mental health had also been challenging at times. After my parents' divorce, my dad found love again with Kathy and they had a son, Reuben, who became the centre of my dad's world. Sadly, his relationship with Kathy didn't last, but my dad's love for his son never wavered.

Even with his health challenges, Dad made it to his 80th birthday, which I went to celebrate with him and Reuben. Dad had moved away from the Midlands in his late 70s, and Mike and I helped him with this.

Dad was thrilled to hear of Sophie's arrival, but sadly they never met. He died only a matter of weeks later. He received hospice care in his local hospital, and the care he received was second to none. I wrote to the hospital to convey my gratitude.

Before he passed away, I stayed in the hospital grounds in the old nurses' quarters, to be near to him, and I am so glad I did. My mum really struggled with this, as she felt he hadn't been there for us so why would I be there for him. But I needed to do it for him and for me.

In the months before his death, we had many conversations about my illness and how I had decided to manage getting better. He was truly interested and wanted to understand, and that meant a lot to me.

In 2019, Mum celebrated her 80th birthday. Her ill health meant travel by plane wasn't possible. However, in the past she had managed to go on a few beautiful cruises with my stepdad John, family, and friends, and it was something that she had really enjoyed. So, she and I decided we would go on a cruise round the Mediterranean.

We travelled by train from Malaga to Barcelona. My mum, by this point, travelled with a portable oxygen machine and had limited mobility. But with the help of some amazing staff in the beautiful train carriage, we did the first leg of the journey without any problems. We stayed overnight in a hotel and could see the cruise ship from our window.

Cruising had never been something I fancied doing, but I went with it for Mum's sake, and with the help of an amazing travel agent Sarah in the UK, all the arrangements were put in place. This included oxygen provision on the cruise, which was the biggest headache to arrange, but made a massive difference to my mum. The suite, the staff, the food, and the experience helped create a truly memorable trip for us both. And there was a lovely butler who would seem to appear just as we needed help with something.

Mum didn't leave the ship until our journey's end at Barcelona. She had hoped to go onshore in Monte Carlo for the Grand Prix, but it involved having to travel into the port on a smaller vessel, which wasn't an option with restricted mobility. We could hear the roar of the cars from way out at sea, though!

I cannot put into words how amazing and important that trip was for both of us, and what incredibly special memories were made. My mum would share about my illness to people she met on board, making me realise how proud she was of me.

2019 also saw us losing our amazing little protector Alfie. He was very poorly and then rallied, and then declined again.

Eventually, we had to make the toughest but kindest decision. Alfie had been with us for 16 years, through the bad times and the good times, and had brought laughter, joy and, most of all, unconditional love for all of us. He used to check on everyone before he went to bed to make sure we were all where we were meant to be.

I got the opportunity to share a very small part of my journey in the collaborative book, *The Girls Who Refused to Quit*, in April 2020, after I had met the publisher, Cassandra Welford, at a fundraising event. The fundraiser was a Summer Ball in aid of The Healing Horse Sanctuary. I was a Trustee at the time, and this amazing event raised much-needed money for the beautiful horses and ponies at the sanctuary.

My Reiki teacher and friend Susie Gessey is also the Founder and Trustee of The Healing Horse Sanctuary, and I have spent many happy and emotional times with her beautiful horses. On one particular day when I was on a Reiki course at the sanctuary, I was honoured to be working with Chester. Chester had needed a forever home, and when he arrived at the sanctuary, he had very visible scars. But I didn't know this.

I went outside my comfort zone and went into the field with the help of two lovely helpers who helped to steady my nerves. I approached Chester and put my hands on his neck to send healing to him. At this point, he moved his body round and I saw all his scars. My own scars from my surgery were still very visible at that time. I received healing from Chester that day; we honoured each other and our scars.

I felt able to share a part of my cancer story with Cassandra's help and support and the other amazing ladies in *The Girls Who Refused to Quit*. I didn't tell anyone, including my girls, that I was part of this project until the day when I needed help with finding suitable clothes and makeup for the online launch. My girls knew that I had wanted to write about my experiences, and they were thrilled when I finally made the decision to write my own book and share my journey.

Due to the pandemic, we didn't manage an in-person book launch for *The Girls Who Refused to Quit,* but the virtual launch was amazing. When my printed copies were delivered, I was so proud of the book and the ladies who had shared their stories. I hand-delivered the book to friends and family that had asked for copies after the launch, and felt proud that I had shared a part of my cancer journey which would hopefully help others.

Each chapter in the book shares a message to the author's younger self. Mine starts with... if I could go back in time and speak to my younger self, I would tell her with great love and honesty not to be so hard on herself.

I sent a copy to my mum in Spain, with a special handwritten message.

My mum didn't understand some of the holistic therapies and treatments I had used to help me not only recover from my cancer surgery and treatment, but also to take care of my general health and wellbeing so that I could continue to live a happy, healthy life. She absolutely wanted that happy, healthy life for me, but didn't really understand some of what I was doing.

Sadly, during the pandemic, we lost the eldest member of our family – my dear mum-in-law Lawrenzina, at the amazing age of 98! This was an incredibly tough time for all the family, and we never got to honour her in the way she would have wanted. There were only ten of us at the graveside, not the beautiful Catholic mass that she would have liked in the church she had attended for over 60 years. My mum-in-law's faith had been her constant support.

Stan's mum and I had enjoyed a relationship that had its highs and lows. She shared with me her amazing curry recipes in the early days, and trusted me to deal with medical appointments and such things for her in later years. I referred to her as Mum, and she was a strong mother figure to me and for the entire family – a woman I greatly admired for her grit and determination.

One of the challenges after serious illness can be anxiety and feelings of fear and isolation. During the pandemic, I think it would be fair to say we all experienced different levels of isolation.

Since my illness, I had come to rely on contact with others as my support to gain a deeper understanding of my health, wellbeing, and healing.

But during the pandemic, I had to come to terms with the fear and anxiety that could sometimes get the better of me. It also highlighted other experiences of feeling incredibly isolated and alone throughout my life. This time allowed me to accept my feelings and to treat myself as I would treat others. I went through a period where I was frightened to go out of the house on my own. However, walking in nature became my therapy, and gradually the walks got longer and allowed me to clear my head and let go of the ridiculous list of things that I was worrying about.

During the time when travel restrictions were in place, my own mum's health deteriorated, and her doctor in Spain provided the necessary documentation for me to travel out to see her. This was at the point when testing was required, along with reams of documentation. I flew out on a flight with 14 other people on the aircraft, plus crew, from a near-empty airport in the UK to an eerily quiet Malaga airport. It was a bizarre experience.

Each time I travelled out to see my mum, we made the most of our time together, leaving her beautiful apartment whenever we could. There were times, though, when a helping hand was needed. Mum had a favourite restaurant where we would go to celebrate our birthdays, and on one occasion we managed to get to our favourite place, but she needed the now ever-present oxygen machine. We got to our table and had a beautiful dinner, but leaving was a whole different ball game. The lift wasn't working, and Mum could not physically manage the stairs. So, with the help of the head waiter, we improvised and used the kitchen lift where all the produce was delivered to and from the kitchen. Not very glamorous, but extremely practical!

In November 2020, after an amazing month-long trip to France and Spain with Mike, where we seemed to be followed by dogs wherever we went, we decided a new four-legged addition to the family was needed. We contacted various rescue centres near where we lived, and they sent through pictures. One particular little girl caught our eye – Dolly, an 18-month-old terrier cross that had come from Romania.

We had been looking during the lockdown and also when the restrictions had lifted. But Mike was very taken by the picture of Dolly and asked if I was able to go the rescue centre and see her. This was arranged, and the next day I met Dolly.

She had come from Romania by truck, wasn't eating, and was petrified of pretty much everything. The lovely guy I met at the rescue centre brought Dolly to a dedicated safe area, and we sat in the rain letting her just be. We took a little bit of food, as at that point she was being fed by hand. She let me feed her a little bit of food, then very, very slowly she started to stretch out from being curled up in a tiny ball. Nearly an hour later, she stretched out enough to tap me on the arm! I just melted at that point, and the connection was made.

I was wearing a purple scarf (I'm rarely without one!), and I left it with Dolly in her bed so that she knew I was coming back for her. Due to Covid restrictions that came into place the following day, we were unable to go back and collect her. But after we had had the necessary checks by the rescue centre, they approved us, and Dolly was delivered to us.

It wasn't the easiest welcome for her, with all of us in masks, and Dolly decided to hide under a huge rhododendron bush in our garden until the lovely chap from the rescue centre retrieved her and we got her into the kitchen.

Dolly, now named Dottie (partly because of the beautiful markings on her paws), has gone from being frightened of everyone and everything, to being a happy, very active, sociable little girl, and we adore her. We surrounded her in love and reassured her, and she is just another bundle of unconditional love!

As I have mentioned before, Mum had her own health problems, and living in Spain meant that she had treatments for her emphysema which were not available in the UK. The warmth of the sun helped her, too, as she couldn't cope with the cold and damp weather here. She was always an incredibly proud lady whose appearance mattered to her a great deal, but as her health deteriorated, even getting dressed in her beautiful clothes became a challenge. Despite the distance between us, I would still chat to Mum every day on the phone, and we checked up on each other in lots of ways.

In November 2021, I decided to challenge myself. For a long time I have wanted to share my story in order to inspire others, but I was stuck in a rut! I had been introduced to Richard McCann on LinkedIn, as Cassandra had been to one of his retreats and raved about it. So, I emailed Richard regarding a place, and he asked why I wanted to attend. In my email, I said I needed to be pushed outside my comfort zone!

This was a three-day retreat in a beautiful hotel in North Yorkshire. If I recall correctly, there were only ten attendees, so not too overwhelming. The weekend was an opportunity to gain experience about storytelling, public speaking, and lots of practical help. It was interactive and petrifying, all at the same time.

We had to stand up at the front of the room and introduce ourselves on the first day. I was shaking, my palms were sweaty, and I just about managed to introduce myself before dashing back to my seat. However, we were up and down from our seats to the front of the room, speaking in front of the other attendees for most of the weekend.

That first day was challenging on so many levels, and I sat in my chair at the end of that initial session, feeling completely and utterly exhausted. After a night's sleep we resumed. Then we had another long day of learning and interaction, with the final presentations to be made on the Sunday. We were all working towards this short presentation, but we had been asked not to share our subject matter before that time.

I was first up on the Sunday, nervous but grateful for everything I had learnt. I had my notes written on an A2 sheet of paper, which was hanging off the edge of the table in front of me, and I had written some of my experiences on sticky labels to signify being labelled. We often label ourselves, but those around us can label us too. I wanted to peel off these labels in a symbolic way during my presentation, but the only problem was they wouldn't stick to the fabric of the dress I was wearing. It didn't go totally to plan, but that's life!

That day was another turning point for me. I shared more of my story, my voice trembled in places, but I did it! Thank you, Richard, for your help and support.

I made another trip out to see my mum in December 2021 and discovered that in the three months since I had last visited her, she had lost three stones in weight. Video calls are amazing, but you don't get to hug and hold your loved ones. And when I hugged my mum that first day of my trip, I just managed to hold back the tears of shock and dismay. Mentally, my mum was still very capable, but the same could definitely not be said for her physical body. During my stay, I helped Mum sort things in her apartment, things that mattered and concerned her, and we managed to make it out of the apartment once for a meal. It was incredibly hard to leave her and return to the UK.

Mike and I celebrated Christmas at home with Sarah, Shammie, Sophie, Georgina, and William, and then with Mike's family. But then in January 2022, things changed again. My relationship with Mike fell to pieces, and we decided to go our separate ways. I still love him, but sometimes you reach a point where you want different things out of life, and that is the stage we had reached. I have been through amazing times and also tough times of loss and ill health, but this loss after 17 years has been incredibly hard. We put our beautiful home on the market and started to pack up our belongings. It was a house move I hadn't anticipated.

Over the past few years, my mum and her deteriorating health had always been in the back of my mind. At one point, many years ago, I had hoped that she would split her time between the UK and Spain. But that decision was taken out of everyone's hands when she was no longer able to fly. As a result, I always made the trips to see her instead.

When I had visited her in the December, we had discussed all sorts of things, including the tough stuff that isn't easy to talk about. Mum made it very clear to me then that she didn't want to die in the hospital where my stepdad had died back in 2008. That was not a slight on the hospital, but more the fact that she wanted to be in her own home, which had been her safe and happy place for over 22 years.

In February, Mum was really struggling, and something happened which resulted in her being admitted to hospital. I am not sure whether that was a mini stroke, a heart attack, or something completely different. After her initial treatment, I think she discharged herself from hospital and made the decision to be at home.

I was incredibly concerned and immediately made arrangements to fly over. I emailed Mum on that Friday to say I would ring her later in the day, then I sorted what I needed to before leaving. When I rang her and explained that I had got a flight and would be with her by lunchtime the next day, we chatted for a while, and she said I was an angel for going over to be with her. Mike took me to the airport, as he had done so many times since my stepdad John died back in 2008.

Mum would always want me to message her to let her know when I was boarding the plane, and again when I arrived at Malaga. So, I sent my usual message and turned my phone off for the flight. But when I arrived at Malaga, I checked my phone and saw she hadn't opened the earlier message.

There were huge delays in passport control and baggage, which took over an hour. Thankfully, I was always collected by the same guy every time I visited, and his younger brother had been waiting patiently for me getting out of the airport.

As we set off for Mum's, she still hadn't responded to the message, and I was getting really concerned. I rang the house, but there was no answer, and I had a strange feeling that is very hard to describe.

There were more delays on the road to Mum's, but as we slowly got nearer to her house, I started to feel more anxious.

When we finally arrived, I immediately knew something was wrong. My mum's dearest friends of many, many years were sitting on the step at the entrance of the walkway to her apartment. I completely lost the plot and began wailing and sobbing.

They explained that her best friend had gone to check on Mum when she hadn't replied to her messages, but it seemed that Mum had died during the night and was lying peacefully in her bed.

There are no words to describe the loss I still feel. My mum and I had our differences over many things over the years, but over the last five years I tried to love, support, and bring as much joy into her life as possible, and I'm very glad I did.

I then had the horrendous task of being the bearer of bad news again. I rang my sister, my daughters, Mike, and then couldn't do any more.

The format for funerals is very different in Spain from the UK. There is usually a cremation within 48 hours, but we needed time for family to be able to fly out from the UK, so we managed to delay the funeral by another day. We needed to write a eulogy, notify family and friends, organise flowers; the list goes on. But you have so little time to make arrangements, unlike here.

I stayed with a friend of Mum's that first night, as I could not be in the apartment. My sister and some of her family arrived on the Sunday. Georgina and the rest of my sister's family arrived on the Monday, and the funeral was on the Tuesday.

I messaged a friend in the UK who is a celebrant, to ask if she had any words of advice for writing the eulogy. She sent me a list of points to cover, which proved invaluable.

My mum had been very private about her life and her achievements, and it's only when someone passes away that you realise you should have asked more questions, taken the time to note down dates, places, and things that were important to her. My sister and I did manage to write her eulogy, and we honoured her as she would have wanted in the same chapel that we honoured her loving husband John, my kind and loving stepdad. We had our words translated into Spanish, so that all those in the chapel could hear more about Mum.

This is where I thank Richard McCann again for his words of wisdom and the part he played in helping me to finally find my voice. I knew I wanted to read my Mum's eulogy, and I did. I hope I made her proud and shared her achievements and what mattered to her.

As I mentioned before, I recently had the opportunity to share a little part of my story in a book called *Beautifully Broken*, and my chapter was called 'Bereavement and Blessings'. We grieve those we have lost, and hope and trust that there are also blessings from these relationships, too.

Chapter: Nine

That brings me to May 2022.

I moved house and started a fresh chapter in a new place.

I also had the opportunity to do something that I had wanted to do since I was lying in a hospital bed back in June 2020! I finally found my voice and shared my story in front of an audience – albeit not a big audience, but one that appreciated my honesty and wished to share my story. Cassandra Welford gave me that opportunity, and I will be forever grateful.

The event was 'The Heart Led Speakers', and all of us who shared our stories that day did so from our hearts. I had been given some guidance in advance by a lovely female speaking coach, but I have always known what I would like to share about my experiences.

I travelled to the venue feeling extremely nervous, but also excited at this opportunity. And I was absolutely outside my comfort zone when I stood up and spoke. Initially, I struggled to get my words out, but then they just flowed – as did the tears in the audience. It was a day of serious highs for all of us who spoke that day. We shared from our hearts, and that is so powerful. The feedback was amazing!

I would like to finish on an amazing high note, as I have shared the highs and the lows of my journey to this point.

In July this year, my youngest daughter Georgina married her best friend William, and I gained another kind and caring son-in-law. It was a spectacular day filled with love, laughter, and tears. So much love had gone into making it a day for all of us to cherish, and we also remembered all our loved ones in spirit, with beautiful photographs and candles, and talked about the good times.

I was overwhelmed by the love I received that day, too. We celebrated the fact that we were all together, and after the experiences of the last few years, I think is fair to say that we all fully appreciated this very, very special time.

I try to take each day as it comes and share the love I have in my heart with others. And I will continue to do that for as long as I possibly can.

When we have the opportunity to reflect, as I have done with this book, it highlights those incredibly low and frightening times, like when I lay in a hospital bed, willing myself to stay alive and keep going with my life. That sheer determination has allowed me to enjoy the incredible times of seeing my beautiful daughters marrying, and the birth of an amazing granddaughter. In my world, there is nothing more precious.

Where do I go from here?

I am still finding my way, but I am proud to announce that by publishing my book, **I have finally found my voice!**

Insights, lessons, therapies, and reflections

I would like to share an insight into my life and my story. I have always wanted to help others, and I have recently been described as a 'humble warrior'. It has taken 54 years for me to acknowledge myself as a Healer.

Part of the journey has been being brave enough to show up as the slightly wacky, Reiki loving, crystal collecting, spiritual soul that I am now.

I am a work in progress. We all are.

But I have learnt a lot, particularly over the last 20 years. And I have learnt that I need to put myself on my list of people I love and care for.

I have studied different types of healing modalities, and I am sure I will learn more.

Gratitude

I sometimes joke that if I listed all the people I am grateful to, the list would stretch the length of my arms. But gratitude is incredibly powerful.

I am grateful to be alive.

I am grateful to my two beautiful daughters for supporting me and making me incredibly proud.

I am grateful to my late husband for teaching me to be independent and strong.

I am grateful to my partner for putting up with me during my illness, my outbursts, and strange requests.

I am grateful to my healing friends who have helped me to heal, learn, and gain confidence.

I am grateful to my mum for showing me strength and determination and respecting my decision to write about my illness.

I am grateful to the dentist who referred me to hospital.

I am grateful to the entire medical team who took care of me.

I am also grateful in a strange way for the times when things did not quite go as planned – in those moments, I really found my own strength and determination.

I am grateful to my family and friends who have always looked out for me and still invited me to celebrations when I looked horrendous!

I am grateful to my beautiful little Jack Russell Alfie (who sadly died in 2020) for protecting me, sleeping at my feet, and checking on us all as we slept.

I am grateful to my gorgeous little Romanian rescue dog Dottie for being my reason to get out of bed on days when I didn't feel like it.

I am grateful for the simple things in life.

I am grateful every day – and that is incredibly powerful!

Self-Care

I have learnt techniques to deal with anxiety and pain.

I am strong, safe, protected, and loved, and I will continue taking good care of myself, my body, my mind, and my spirit, in the ways that work best for me.

My healing journey since my cancer surgery has been one of discovery and learning.

Self-care is vital, and it's sometimes when you reach your absolute lowest point that you realise its importance.

I maintain my health and wellbeing with regular Reflexology, Reiki, and Acupuncture sessions, along with regular supplements and herbal medicine.

Without my health, how can I enjoy making memories with my family and friends, travelling to new places and others I know and love, and most importantly sharing my love of life?

Speaking up for yourself

Now, you might think that this is an obvious one for me, having read about my cancer journey.

From a very early age, though, I was taught to do as I was told. That, of course, is fine if you are also helped and guided to speak up for yourself. But this has been a tough lesson for me.

Some of my experiences as a youngster were brushed aside, when I tried to explain about being abused, bullied, and other tough experiences. I feel that some of that was related to others not wanting to hear unpleasant things.

I have read many books over the last ten years that talk about trauma, and how our bodies react to stress and trauma. I suffered various spells of ill health before my cancer diagnosis, but I do feel that there was a connection with me being 'shut up' lots of times over many years.

Part of me allowed others to silence me, and that is something I regret. We all have opinions, ideas, and things we need to say and express in different ways. I fought to get my voice back, literally, sounding out the letters of the alphabet and saying numbers to regain my ability to speak. I had to learn to eat and swallow again.

In the last ten years, there have also been times when I have literally bitten my tongue and not expressed my true feelings. However, writing about my experiences is a chance to share my truth and my knowledge. I hope my story has helped you gain insight, but most of all inspiration to speak up for yourself and take care of yourself. Everything I have shared has been written to inspire and uplift you with love.

Helpful techniques, healing modalities,
and doing what makes you happy!

Journal writing and spreadsheets

I have always written things down, from a basic shopping list to that becoming my only means of communication when I couldn't speak. Sometimes we just need to write things down so that they are not going round and round in our heads. A pen and paper have been invaluable for me.

I might not like creating spreadsheets, but having them during my recovery was invaluable. They enabled not only me to keep an eye on what medication I was on or what I was eating, but also helped those taking care of me at home.

Your notebook or journal is yours, and it's a place where you can empty your head and heart of emotions and thoughts – good and bad.

I also use my notebooks to acknowledge how grateful I am for my life, my experiences, and to plan what I want to do next. I have had various times in my life where planning really wasn't something I felt I could do. After my husband's death, I didn't feel I could plan or look forward more than a couple of days at a time. But it really helps to have something to look forward to. That might be something like meeting up with a friend or writing a bucket list. I still have places I want to see in the world and things I want to learn.

Why not treat yourself to a beautiful notebook and pen? You can share how you feel without judgement, and if you want to share what you have written, then that's up to you.

Counselling

A non-judgemental listening ear. During our lives, we have good times and bad times – it is part of life. You might look around you and think everyone around you has it all sorted – but don't be fooled.

My first experience of counselling was after the death of my husband, when I was just 34. I had taken care of him to the best of my ability and with great love, and I was completely devastated when he died. My focus was then on taking care of our daughters.

My doctor at the time recommended I go for a six-week course of counselling – one hour a week for six weeks. It was good to talk to someone who had no prior knowledge of me and my experiences, and the lovely lady I met was supportive and kind. That first experience was a positive one, and I think that is one of the reasons I have been happy to go for counselling again when I have needed to.

I think one of the most beneficial things about counselling is that it is a safe space to be heard without judgement, and also to gain much-needed guidance when things are tough. Sometimes you can feel differently about a situation when you are supported and have time to make sense of how you really feel.

When you are struggling, the input of a kind and compassionate person who will allow you to say how you feel and not judge you can be an opportunity to make peace with different situations or traumas you have experienced.

Affirmations

Words are powerful. The words we read or hear can change how we feel in a second. Also, the words we tell ourselves. I have a plaque on my desk that my youngest daughter gave me.

'You are braver than you believe, stronger than you seem, and smarter than you think.'

When I first received my diagnosis, I asked my friend Susie if she could suggest an affirmation that I could use. She suggested: 'I am healed, and I am free to be me.' That is one line of words that I have probably said out loud or in my head a thousand times in the last ten years.

Perhaps one of my own lessons has been the importance of speaking kindly to myself. I have a tendency to be very hard on myself, but I've learnt that no longer serves me. I wouldn't talk to my friends like that, so why would I continue to talk to myself that way?

If you want to find out more on the subject, Louise Hay wrote many books on Affirmations, as have many other health and wellbeing writers.

Before I go to sleep, I usually write in my journal. It is a chance to review my day, feel gratitude for everything, and hopefully settle for a good night's sleep.

Some of my affirmations are:

I am well

I am strong

I am loving

I am loved

I am kind

I am compassionate

I am safe

I am protected

I am grateful

Sometimes in life we need to remind ourselves that we are all of these.

Having had cancer can leave its mark on you, both physically and emotionally. For me, it has left an element of anxiety. I realise that I have had periods of high anxiety and stress throughout my life, and I am doing my best to overcome this.

I am doing the best I can!

Acupuncture

Acupuncture forms part of the ancient practice of Traditional Chinese Medicine, and has been used in China for over 2500 years. Very fine needles are inserted into specific points on the body to enable the optimum flow of Qi for the person. Qi (essentially the life-force) can be impacted by many factors, for example, our work, the environment, pathogens and climate, our ancestry, relationships, and our constitution.

Five Element acupuncture is based on a model of dynamic balance between the Elements (Water, Wood, Fire, Earth, Metal) reflected in the cycle of the seasons (Winter, Spring, Summer, Late Summer, Autumn). It seeks to support each person on their unique path through life, physically, mentally, emotionally, and spiritually.

Hypnotherapy

Hypnotherapy is one of the most natural forms of therapy that, with the consent of the individual, utilises their own innate resources to make positive changes for themselves, both psychologically and physically.

Hypnosis is an 'altered state of consciousness' similar to a sleepy dozing or daydreaming state where, with the help of the therapist, the mind is more receptive to making positive changes for the person.

Hypnotherapy is a safe and effective form of therapy that has proven to work with many different psychological and physical ailments. When a person is in a hypnotherapy session, the therapist helps them to achieve a more relaxed state where they are still in control and 'aware' of what is taking place. In this altered state of consciousness, the unconscious/subconscious part of a person's mind becomes more receptive to acceptance of suggestion, in order to effect positive change, psychologically or physically, for the individual.

Hypnotherapy is a fantastic tool for releasing past trauma on a physical, mental, emotional, and spiritual level. By tapping into the subconscious mind, we can unlock and let go of many non-serving thoughts, feelings, memories, and energies that we may not even be aware are impacting on our daily thoughts and actions.

Letting go of 'old patterns', creating and repeatedly walking through new neural pathways, leads to lasting positive growth and frees us up to reach our fullest potential.

Tapping, or Emotional Freedom Technique (EFT)

Tapping provides relief from chronic pain, emotional problems, disorders, addictions, phobias, post-traumatic stress disorder, and physical diseases. While tapping is newly set to revolutionise the field of health and wellness, the healing concepts that it's based upon have been in practice in Eastern medicine for over 5,000 years. Like acupuncture and acupressure, Tapping is a set of techniques which utilise the body's energy meridian points. You can stimulate these meridian points by tapping on them with your fingertips – literally tapping into your body's own energy and healing power.

Your body is more powerful than you can imagine… filled with life, energy, and a compelling ability for self-healing. With Tapping, you can take control of that power.

Usui Reiki

Reiki (ray-key) is Japanese for 'universal life energy' and is also a word used to describe a system of natural healing. This tradition was founded by Mikao Usui in the early 20th century, and evolved as a result of his research, experience, and dedication. When this energy flows uninterrupted, there is balance and harmony within and around us, and we experience a sense of wellbeing.

There are many variations of Reiki, but in essence Reiki treatments can help the body emotionally and spiritually. It is a tradition that is open to any belief system. Reiki can be used alongside other conventional or complementary treatments, and often helps to provide emotional support during recovery.

Angelic Reiki

Angelic Reiki is a complete system of hands-on energy healing which was channelled from the Archangel Metatron through Kevin Core in 2003, and it has since continued to evolve with the new energies affecting our planet and human consciousness. Since 2001, the vibration of the Angelic Kingdom has merged with Earth and Humanity in a way not experienced for millions of years; hence the upsurge in all things angelic. Angels are gifting Humanity with the knowledge of their own Divinity, and there are many people contacting and channelling this energy. One of the purest forms of this is Angelic Reiki – a healing modality that connects us with our own Divinity, our Higher Self.

Crystal Reiki Therapy

This therapy enables the therapist to use Reiki healing energy with the gifts of Mother Nature in the form of crystals. This can be another beautiful soothing therapy for body, mind, and soul.

Aromatherapy

Aromatherapy is the practice of using essential oils for therapeutic benefit and has been used for centuries. When inhaled, the scent molecules in essential oils travel from the olfactory nerves directly to the brain, and especially impact the amygdala – the emotional centre of the brain. Essential oils can be used in very subtle ways to bring calm, not only to a person but to the environment they are in.

Sound healing

A beautiful use of sound in sound healing or sound baths is amazing. You get comfortable – usually snuggled under blankets – and let the sound vibrations created by beautiful gongs, singing bowls, and other instruments, travel through your body and surround you. There are certain people who cannot have this treatment for health reasons, e.g., pregnancy, heart conditions, or some forms of mental illness.

Massage and Lymphatic drainage

There are many, many different types of massage, and there are practitioners who are trained to help people after a cancer diagnosis.

Pathogenics

Pathogenics is the practice of detecting and clearing pathogens in the body, addressing health conditions at the root, accurately, efficiently, remotely, without the use of supplements, dietary changes, or any additional treatments or blood tests. As pathogens are cleared, you begin to heal.

Exercise

I have never been a great fan of exercise in the form of running, going to the gym, or classes. Maybe I never found one that I felt comfortable with. Since my illness, though, I have tried different forms of yoga and Tai Chi. Walking is what works for me, and our beautiful dog Dottie has been my buddy, making sure I now walk every day. We all need to find what works for us as individuals, but I would just suggest you try different things to support your body, and the people you meet can also help and inspire you.

And for my final words...

I am healed, I am strong, and I deserve to be heard.

Feel free to use this affirmation to remind you that **your** voice always deserves to be heard.

With love and gratitude for taking the time to read my story.

Kate xxx

Reference Section

These are just some of the books which I have used during my healing journey. In my experience, you may feel drawn to a particular book or subject. Just go with it.

Aloe Vera, Nature's Silent Healer, by Alasdair Barcroft & Dr Audun Myskja

Heal Your Body, by Louise Hay

Crystal Power, Crystal Healing, The Complete Handbook, by Michael Gienger

The Crystal Bible 1 & 2, by Judy Hall

Reiki for Life, by Penelope Quest

Brenda's Easy-to-Swallow Cookbook, by Brenda Brady

Why Woo-Woo Works, by David R Hamilton Ph.D.

Your Life in Colour: Empowering Your Soul, with Dougall Fraser

Dying To Be Me, by Anita Moorjani

The Tapping Solution Book, by Nick Ortner

Useful Websites

https://www.mouthcancerfoundation.org/

https://www.thetappingsolution.com/what-is-eft-tapping/

https://www.macmillan.org.uk/

https://www.headspace.com/meditation

About the Author

Kate, who lives in Shropshire, has been described as loving, kind, strong, compassionate, and resilient. An authentic, humble, and brave warrior. Kate's precious family, friends, and fellow practitioners are what make up her world. She has a passion for complementary therapies, sharing her knowledge and skills in many different ways.

Being in nature is key, and particularly enjoying the beautiful Shropshire countryside with her little dog, Dottie.

Kate has been on an enlightening journey which has culminated in her becoming an aromatherapist, Reiki Master, Infinite Energy Healer, and author.

Kate's mission is to be a beacon of light and to inspire others on their journey.

Connect with Kate

kate@scattergoodtherapies.com
www.scattergoodtherapies.com
Instagram: katefernandez2913
LinkedIn: Kate Fernandez

Kate's Books

Kate has contributed with chapters in 'The Girls Who Refused to Quit' and also 'Beautifully Broken'

Signed copies are available to purchase via Kate's website.

Lightning Source UK Ltd.
Milton Keynes UK
UKHW021839081222
413617UK00009B/300

9 781739 097080